THE BEST 7 DAY GREEN SUPERFOOD SMOOTHIE CLEANSE GUIDE

FOR DETOX, HEALING AND WEIGHT LOSS

WITH 3 WEEK MEAL PLAN, 56 RECIPES & MORE..

MARIA TARNEV - WYDRO, HD

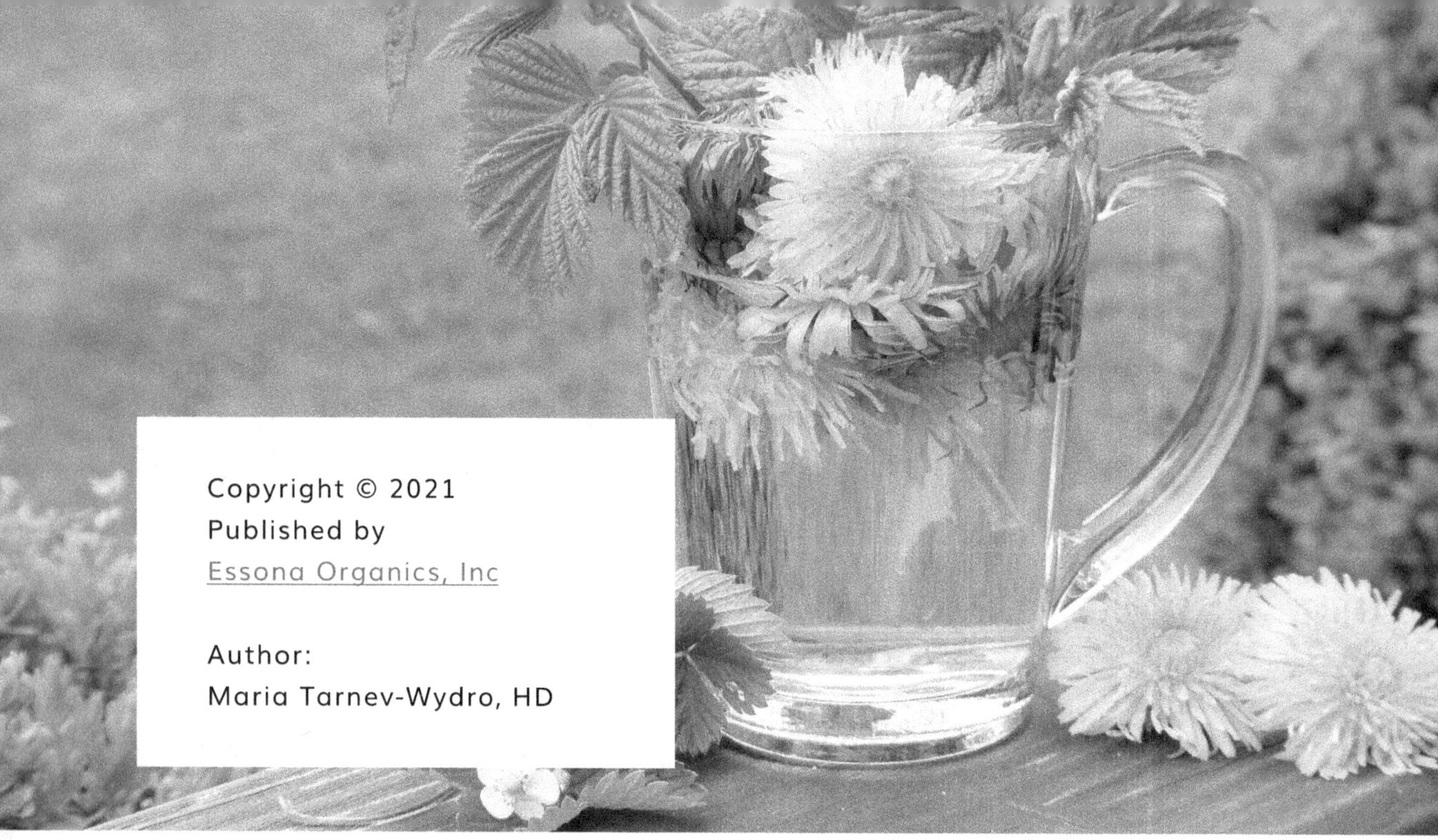

Disclaimer
The author of this book is not a medical doctor. As a health researcher, the author has spent over 20 years investigating the true cause of disease. This book is based on discoveries made by leading researchers which has been compiled from books, scientific papers, medical reports, scientific journals, and ground breaking studies from leading universities and advanced medical research institutions. The author also includes observations of the various treatments developed and practiced by doctors from around the world as well as her own experience and experience gained from her practice.

Before beginning any health program you should consult a licensed health care professional and be monitored throughout the entire process. This book is not intended to provide medical advice, diagnose illness, or in any way attempt to practice medicine. It is educational only and is not intended to replace personal medical care from a licensed health care professional. Doing anything recommended or suggested in this book must be done at your own risk. Neither the publisher nor author takes any responsibility for any adverse consequences to any person reading or following the information in this book.

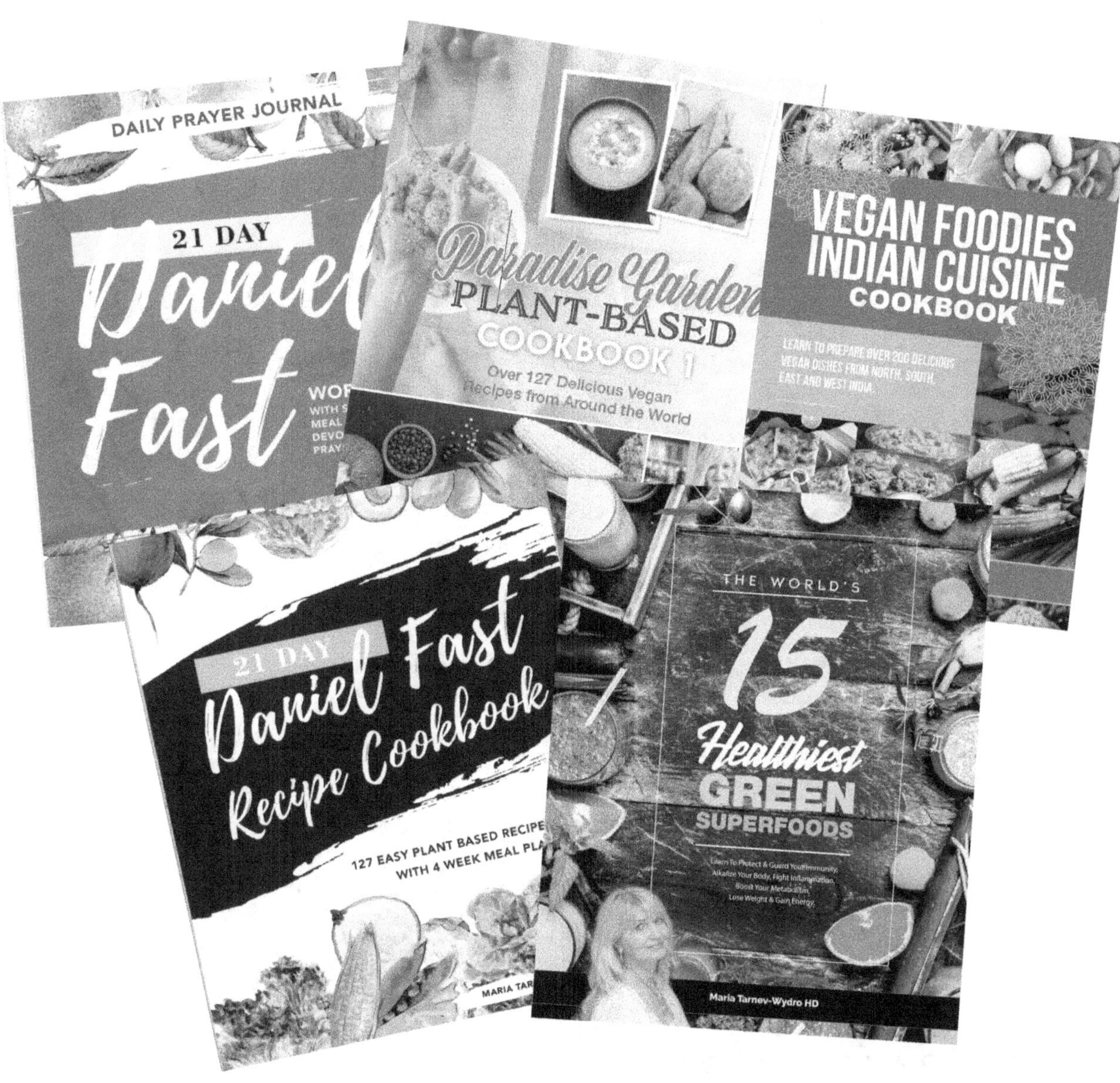

The World's 15 Healthiest Green Superfoods
Vegan Foodies Indian Cuisine Cookbook
Paradise Garden Plant-Based Cookbook 1
21 Day Daniel Fast Workbook and Daily Prayer Journal
21 Day Daniel Fast Recipe Cookbook

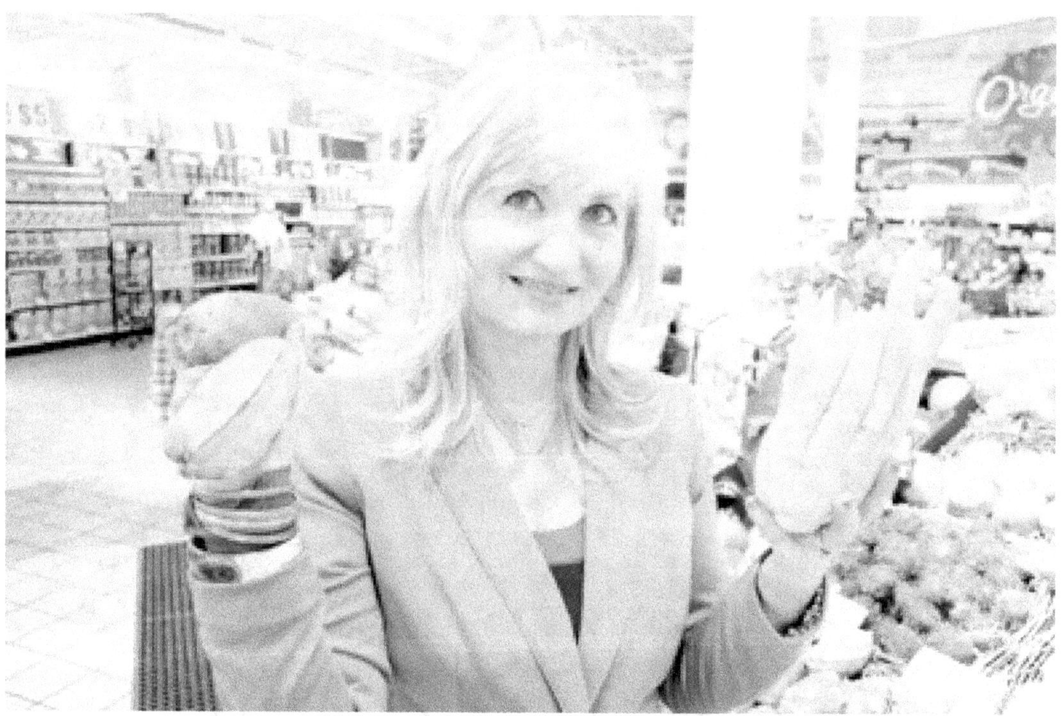

Maria Tarnev-Wydro, HD, is a Homeopathic Doctor, Health and Wellness Coach, mother of 3 children, wife, and the founder of Essona Organics. Her mission is to encourage people to live a healthy, mindful life with purpose. Maria has written several books about faith, health, nutrition, wholistic beauty, healthy cooking and healing.
She loves to share her knowledge and 25 years experience about herbal healing, wholesome diets, cleansing and detox, prayer and fasting and other alternative methods to help those with health issues.

"I look forward to working with you to unlock your true health and wellness!"

Maria Tarnev-Wydro, HD, BSc, Author of several books about health, cooking and faith. She is available to speak at trade shows, groups and organizations.
Founder and President of Essona Organics and DanielFast.org.

www.essona.com

HOW GREEN SUPERFOODS CHANGED MY LIFE - MY STORY

Several years ago, I was diagnosed with an auto-immune disorder (fibromyalgia) and digestive issues. The pain and symptoms made it very difficult to function on a daily basis. I was battling with muscle pain, chronic fatigue, digestive problems and flu-like symptoms. I also had continual weight gain and acid reflux. My severe digestive issues left me with very few food choices.

My dilemma was; how to eat high nutrition foods that were easily digestible and would not trigger my symptoms. I began doing a lot of research about nutrition, and utilizing my knowledge as a Homeopathic Doctor, I came up with a plan to help my body heal. I knew I needed high nutrition foods to build my immune system blended with foods that would help me heal. My research kept pointing me toward Green Superfoods.

The next thing I did was to purchase and evaluate several of the leading "greens" powders on the market and I found out a few things:

- Most of the powders contained powdered vegetables that I can buy fresh at the store.
- Many contained cheap fillers in order to make their product appear larger. Several of them did not mix well in water.
- They all seemed to have a "grassy" taste. From unpleasant to downright horrible.

I would have to make my own. My goal was to formulate a blend that would contain the most powerful functional Green Superfoods, organic and pure, without any fillers, and a good taste so I would look forward to drinking it. It also had to mix well in plain water, be easily digestible and readily absorbable. After much research, trial and error, I finally had a blend that satisfied all the criteria, but I still had one more step. In addition to using it daily myself, I gave it to others to try it and give me their honest feedback. I received much encouraging feedback, made a few small adjustments in the formula and Power Shot Greens Superfood blend was born! **MIX, SHAKE AND DRINK.** Since then, we have had the honor and privilege of helping thousands of people on their journey to improved health and vitality.

Maria Tarnev-Wydro, HD, BSc.

CONTENTS

WELCOME TO THE 7 DAY
GREEN SUPERFOOD SMOOTHIE CLEANSE

Welcome to your 7-Day Green Superfood Smoothie Cleanse! If you're looking for increased energy, to shave some pounds, improved mental clarity and an overall improvement in your health, you've come to the right place.

In this 7 Day Green Superfood Smoothie Cleanse program, you'll learn everything you need to know about how to do a cleanse safely and effectively. This book will not only provide valuable information but will also take you by the hand, step-by-step, and guide you through all phases of the cleanse. The concept behind the program is simple. We give you daily meal plans, weekly shopping lists and nutritional information for each recipe to ensure your success.

All you have to do is follow the program.

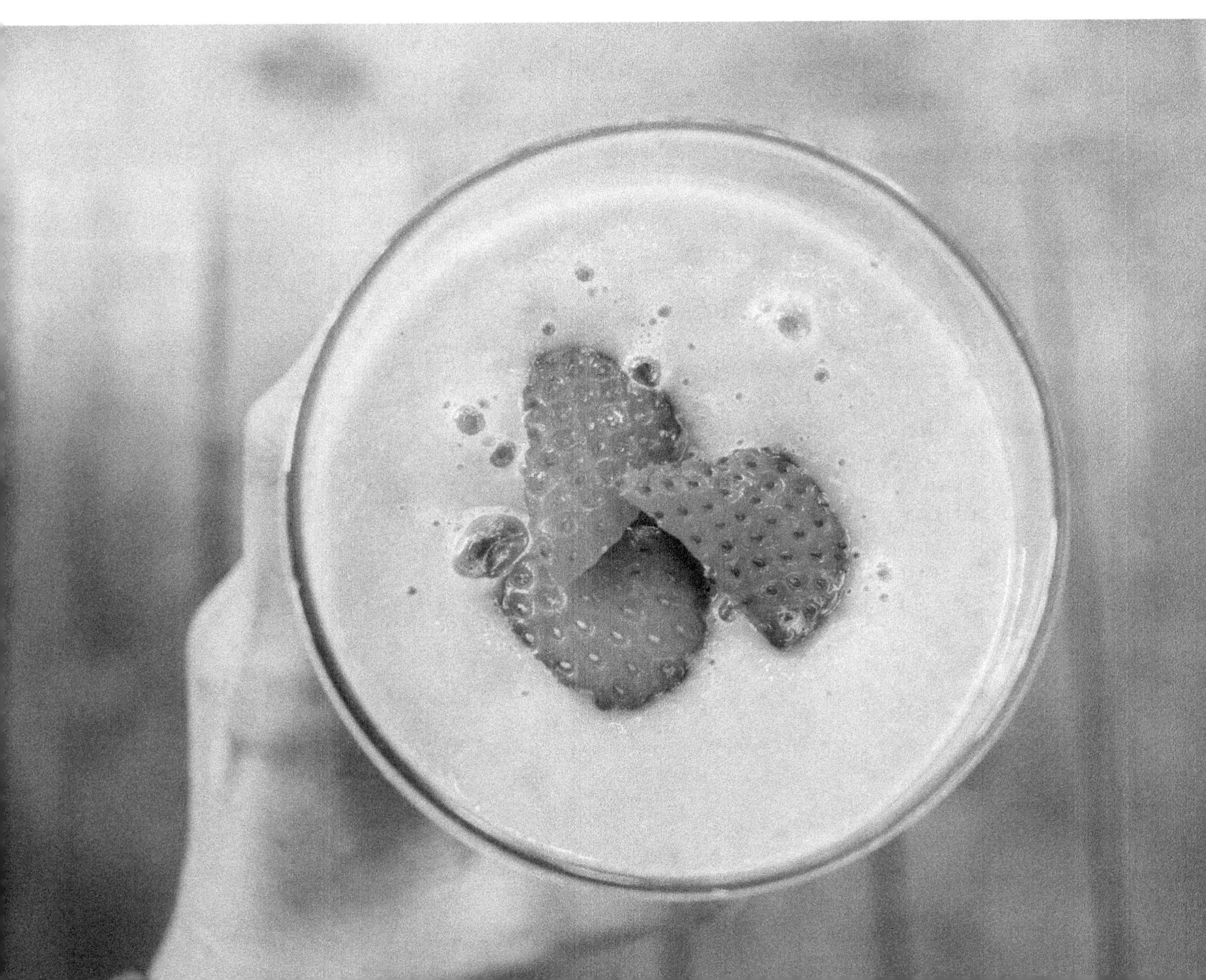

WHAT IS THE DIFFERENCE BETWEEN 'CLEANSING' AND 'DETOXING'?

There is a lot of information available about cleansing and detoxing. Let's take a moment to explain the difference. The words cleansing and detoxifying are often used interchangeably. While there is some overlap in the processes, they are actually distinct actions that happen within your body.

You do a cleanse (modify your diet) in order to allow your body to detoxify. 'Detoxification' primarily occurs in your liver. Certain nutrients, vitamins and minerals are necessary in order for your liver to convert toxins from fat-soluble compounds into water-soluble compounds in order for them to be excreted from your body via urine, feces, breath and sweat. Green Superfoods can provide these necessary nutrients, vitamins and minerals. They are absolutely essential in allowing your liver to do its job efficiently.

WHY DO YOU NEED TO DETOXIFY?

Though our bodies are detoxing continuously, sometimes we need to give it a little assistance. In the US alone, over 84,000 chemicals have been approved by the FDA. The vast majority of these have not undergone safety testing. We are constantly exposed to these chemicals in our homes, our cars, our clothing, the food we eat, the water we drink, even the air we breathe. Our livers are often overwhelmed and cannot keep up.

When this happens, your body uses its innate wisdom to protect itself and stores these toxins away in a safe place, namely, your fat cells. This is one reason why some people have a hard time losing weight. Your body does not want to liberate the toxins if there are not enough resources to detoxify and eliminate them. This is why it's critical that elimination pathways (urine, feces, sweat) are open before embarking on a cleanse. This program will support your liver so your body can detoxify efficiently and allow your body to run at optimum level.

You will also lose weight naturally.

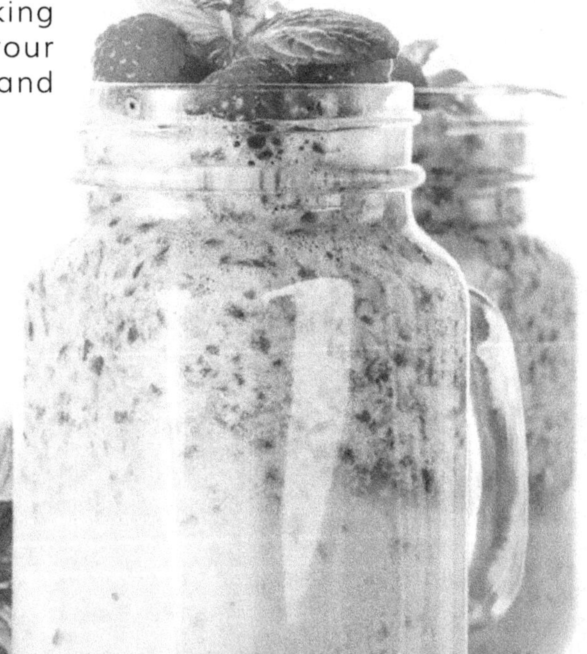

HOW DO YOU KNOW IF YOU NEED TO DETOX?

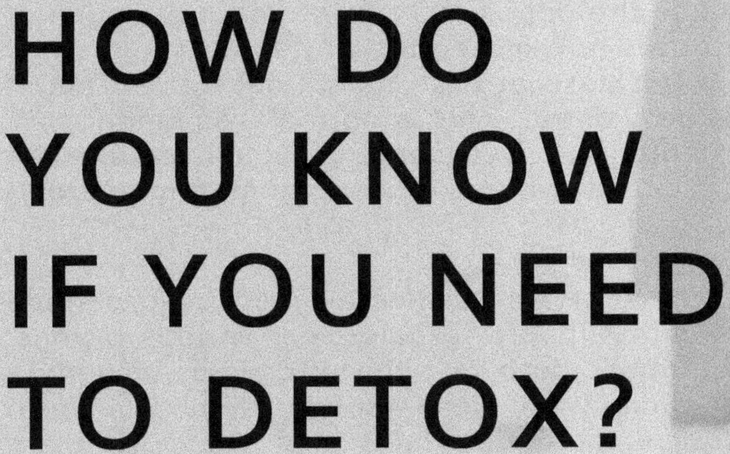

Here are some signs that it's time to start a detox program.

DETOX IF YOU EXPERIENCE:

- Unexplained fatigue
- Sluggish elimination
- Irritated skin
- Allergies
- Menstrual problems
- Bloating

- Mental confusion
- Insomnia
- Constipation
- Chronic Inflammation
- Anxiety, Depression
- Puffy eyes or bags under the eyes

THE SCIENCE BEHIND DETOX

PHYSIOLOGIC

The main physiological change taking place while you detox is in the liver. During this time, the liver finally has the opportunity to be more effective at its job of turning unwanted substances into material that can be excreted by the body. You might experience a backlash at first, as in your system might feel and look a little off before it gets better. This is normal; remember that it's cleansing time. Within approximately two weeks though, you'll begin to see improvements. This will include changes to your skin, hair, mood and energy.

METABOLIC RESPONSES

Speaking in terms of human biochemistry, detoxification can be described as a detailed in and out process with supporting help from various organs. This refers primarily to specific metabolic pathways that processes unwanted substances and prepares them for elimination. This metabolic detox involves a series of enzymes that help neutralize contaminants. It then transports them to secretory organs (like the liver or kidneys), so that they can be removed from the body. This type of detoxification is sometimes called xenobiotic metabolism, because it is the primary mechanism for ridding the body of xenobiotics (foreign substances to the body).

DETOXIFICATION PHASES

There are three phases in the detox process that purifies our entire system. Your liver is the main detoxifying organ in your body and over time, can become sluggish from too much caffeine, alcohol, medications, pesticides, poor food choices, etc. and may need to be detoxified in order to restore it to peak performance. Ridding your body of excess toxins is very important to ensure you do not enter into a state of auto-intoxication because this can be the root cause of all sorts of illnesses.

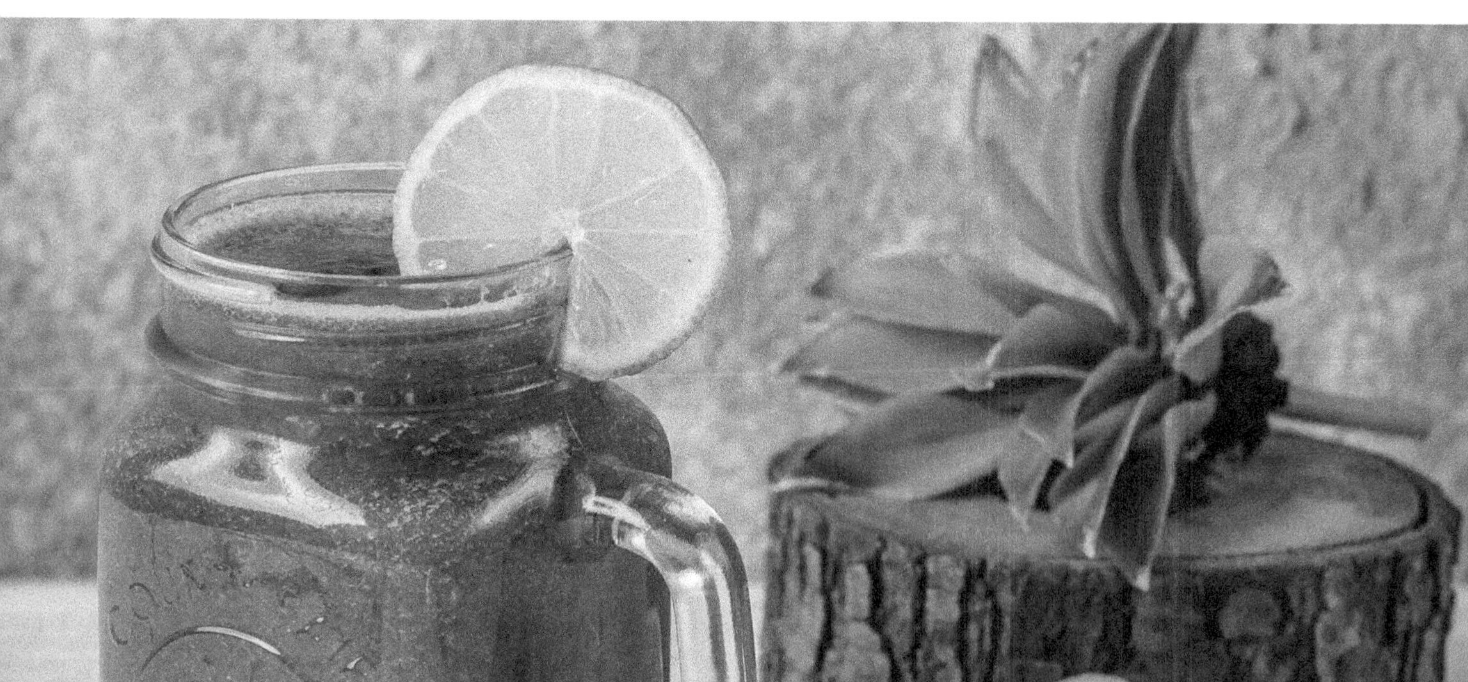

IN PHASE 1: your liver uses a group of enzymes known as cytochrome P 450 to emulsify toxins and break them down and change them from fat soluble to water soluble substances. It is in phase 1 that free radicals are produced which, if excessive, can damage the liver cells. Antioxidant substances, which we can obtain from our food, reduce the damage caused by these free radicals. If, on the other hand, antioxidants are absent, toxic substances become much more dangerous. The best antioxidants to take daily to support your Phase 1 detoxification pathways are antioxidants made from whole foods. In this phase, your liver needs a vast supply of nutrients (Superfoods) to help support it to do the job efficiently.

PHASE 2: is called the conjugation pathway. In this phase the substances are converted to a non-toxic form and are readied to be excreted.

PHASE 3: Once the contaminants are converted to water soluble form, they are excreted from your body via urine, stool and/or perspiration.
Cleansing and detox, while supporting your liver with Superfoods, will optimize this entire process immediately and for the near future. You can always repeat the process as often as you need.

BENEFITS OF DETOXIFICATION

So, what can detox do for me? You ask yourself.
A detox program can help your body's natural cleansing process by:
* Providing a resting period for the organs during fasting stages
* Stimulating the liver to remove contaminants
* Promoting the action of elimination organs (intestines, kidneys, and skin)
* Improving blood circulation
* Refueling the body with healthy nutrients

HOW TO SUPPORT YOUR ORGANS OF ELIMINATION

The liver, kidneys, lungs, intestines and skin are the main organs of elimination. These organs work together to ensure that our body is able to survive in an ever-demanding environment. Because they continuously work hard it is essential that we support these organs. Here are a few easy suggestions of how this can be achieved: Increase your water intake, exercising to make you sweat, regular sweating in a sauna, steam room, hot bath, Jacuzzi will promote release of toxins, practice Intermittent Fasting (IF) and use detox aids as discussed later in this book.

WHAT IS THE CONNECTION BETWEEN FASTING, DETOX & FAT LOSS?

Most people think that losing weight is strictly about reducing or burning calories. As such, it's common for people to believe that if they just restrict calories, they'll lose weight. This may work for a very short time, but it is not an effective long-term strategy. There is much more to losing weight than just restricting calories. However, when done appropriately and in the right context, fasting can be an effective adjunct to a weight loss protocol.

Since the dawn of man, people have been fasting. Before the advent of trains, planes, and refrigerators, food scarcity was a real thing (and still is in many parts of the world). Fasting due to lack of resources was common. You can also find religious, spiritual and political practices of fasting across the globe.

Though fasting can be uncomfortable, it turns out there is significant benefit that goes beyond weight loss.When you fast for more than 12 hours, you activate something called autophagy. Autophagy is the process of 'cellular cleanup' that happens when the body is in a fasted state. The outcome is reduced inflammation, cellular protection, enhanced immune function, weight loss, and many other health benefits.

When you eat frequently, your body has a steady source of glucose to use for energy production. When you extend your overnight fast to longer than 12 hours, your body uses up most of its stored sugar (glycogen). At this time, it reverts to burning fat for fuel instead of glucose. Because it's tapping into its fat stores, there is potential for stored toxins to be liberated. As long as this is done slowly and elimination is functioning optimally, detoxification and fat loss will occur simultaneously.

The thought of fasting can be painful for some people. Thankfully, you don't have to go without food for days on end. There are many approaches to fasting, and most people can find a method that works well for their lifestyle and biochemistry.

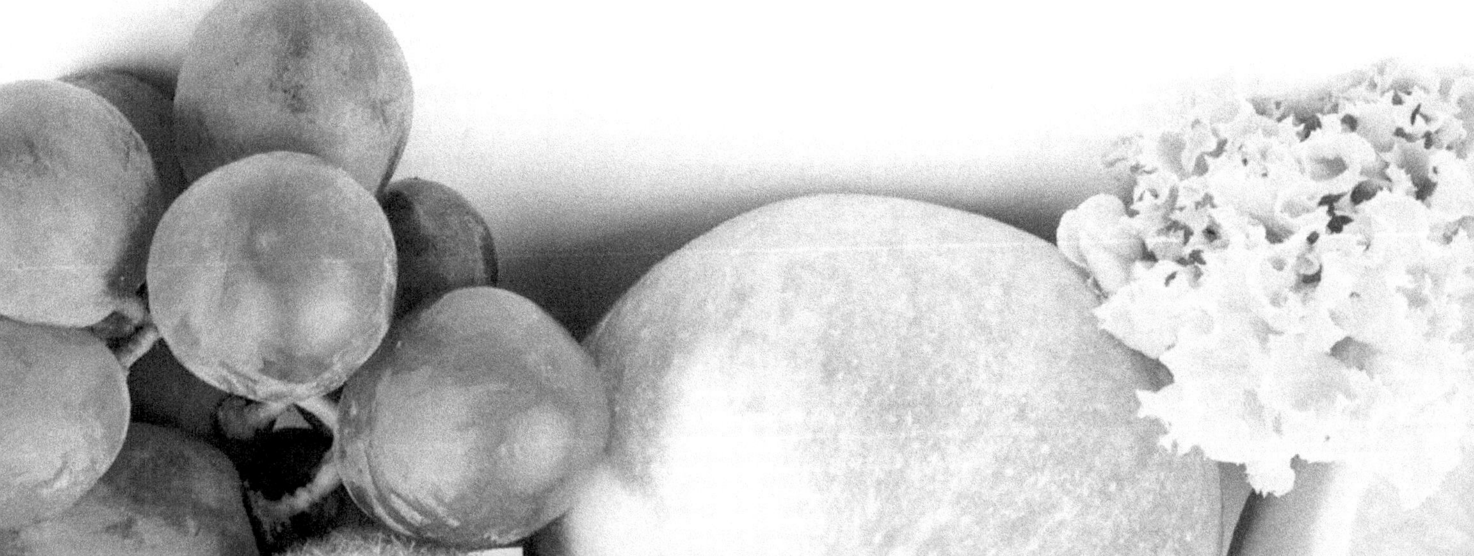

THE MOST POPULAR TYPES OF FASTING

ABSOLUTE FAST :

- 24 HR. FAST: This is the basic 24 hour fast where you consume nothing but water for 24 hours. Clean, filtered water is imperative.

- 3 DAY FAST: This is the basic 3 day fast where you consume nothing but water for 3 days.

PARTIAL FAST :

- LIQUID FAST: A liquid partial fast you're allowed juices or smoothies in addition to water. Durations vary.

- GREEN SMOOTHIE FAST: This type of fasting includes consuming only vegetables blended into a smoothie. Small amounts of fruits or juices may be allowed.

- JUICE FAST: This type of fast allows juiced vegetables or fruits only. The difference between a juice and smoothie fast is the fiber. Blended vegetables will retain their fiber content while juices do not.

- MONO-FAST: A mono-fast requires the dieter to eat only one food for an extended period of time. For example: eating only bananas, or potatoes, or apples, etc.

- 21 DAY DANIEL FAST: It is whole foods vegan partial fast for 21 days. (See 21 Day Daniel Fast Workbook, also by Maria.)

- RAW FOOD FAST: This type of fast consists of eating nothing but raw food. The premise is that cooked food has been denatured and void of all enzymes and vital energy. This 'dead' food is hard to digest and lowers a person's energy field. Typical food choices of a raw food diet include any raw vegetables and fruit, along with soaked and sprouted nuts, seeds, and some legumes.

INTERMITTENT FASTING

Intermittent Fasting (IF) is the practice of cycling between times of fasting and eating normally. Instead of fasting 'now and then,' you practice times of fasting regularly throughout the week. IF has become very popular over the last few years. With the amount of scientific research behind it, it's no wonder. IF has been shown to help with metabolism, weight management, cardiovascular health, inflammation, cognitive issues, and much more. There are several different methods to IF; they range from simply delaying your breakfast, to fasting for a full 24 hours. Let's take a look at several options.

16/8 METHOD
Fast for 18 hours per day, and eat for 6.
This is similar to the 12/12 method, but you're shortening your 'feeding window' to only 8 hours. For most people, this means not eating breakfast, and only consuming two meals per day.
For example: Eat your first meal at 12 noon, eat dinner at 7pm, and take your last bite of food by 8pm. Don't consume any calories until 12noon the next day.

18/6
Fast for 18 hours per day, and eat for 6.

20/4 Method
Fast for 20 hours per day, and eat for 4.
This method can be a little trickier for some, but many people find they enjoy the freedom of not having to think about food except one time per day. In the 20/4 method, your 'feeding window' is only four hours. For most people, this means eating one substantial meal per day. The timing depends on your schedule and preference, but many people choose to have a large dinner.
As an example, you can begin eating at 4pm and finish all caloric intake by 8pm. This allows for a nice casual dinner, allows you to slow down, enjoy your food, have conversations with friends, and be mindful of your eating practices.

ALTERNATE DAY FASTING
This method of fasting has been studied specifically for weight loss and cholesterol benefits with some encouraging results. As you're fasting for a full 24-hours, you may find it more challenging, especially if you have blood sugar handling issues. Only attempt this method after you have experience with something like the 16/8 method.

Here is how it works:
- Choose which days of the week to fast. They should not be consecutive days. You may want to avoid weekends due to social engagements.
- Eat normally as you would on the first day of the week, say that's Sunday.

- Stop eating anything after the dinner meal. (That means no calories via food or beverages.) Let's say you take your last bit of food at 7:00 pm.
- On Monday, fast all day until 7:00 pm. You may have a dinner meal after 7:00 pm.
- On Tuesday, eat as you normally would, but stop eating again at 7:00 pm. You may have no calories past 7:00.
- On Wednesday, fast all day, until 7:00pm.
- You get the idea. Keep fasting during the day every other day and eat as you normally would on the other days. As mentioned above this method can be quite powerful for weight loss.

5:2 METHOD

Otherwise known as 'The Fast Diet', this method involves choosing two days per week where you consume only 25% of your daily caloric needs. This generally translates to approximately 400-600 calories depending on your sex, body size, and energy expenditure. On the other five days, you eat as you normally would.

Here's an example of how it works:
- Choose which two days of the week you will reduce your calories. They should not be consecutive days. Let's say you choose Tuesday and Friday.
- On your 'fasting' days, Tuesday and Friday, consume only 400-600 calories. Make sure the foods you consume are good quality whole foods, not processed or junk foods.
- On Sunday, Monday, Wednesday, Thursday and Saturday, eat as you normally would.
- Be consistent. You change the days of the week you choose to fast, but the more consistency you have, the easier it will become, and the more benefits you will see.

YOUR OWN METHOD

There are not rules to fasting. If there are other methods that meet your needs and are more amendable to your lifestyle, then go for it. Here are some ideas:

- Every week, fast one day per week
- Each month, fast for one specific day.
- Once per month, fast for an entire weekend.
- Reduce your total caloric intake one day per week.
- If you feel well, skip a meal if it seems like a good idea.
- Plan out weekend fasts each time the season's change to prepare the body for the transition.

Examine each IF method to identify which is best for you and your lifestyle. Consider which method would fit your personal lifestyle. Start slowly and work your way into longer fasts if it feels appropriate for you.

WHAT ARE SUPERFOODS?

Before we explain Superfoods, let's talk about the different types of foods. There are 3 basic categories of foods available today.

LEVEL 1 FOODS - PROCESSED FOODS

These are the processed, boxed, canned, instant "foods" found lining the middle aisles of your local grocery store. Also included in this category would be pre-prepared foods from the supermarket as well as restaurant fast foods. These foods are usually high in sugar, salt, high fructose corn syrup, colorants, MSG, GMO's, artificial flavors, unhealthy fats, preservatives and are low in fiber, nutrients and enzymes. These "foods" weaken your immune system making you susceptible to viruses, colds, high blood pressure, diabetes and other

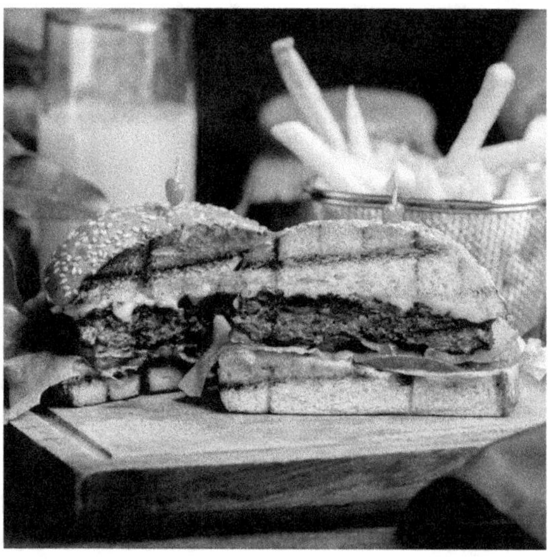

chronic illnesses. Most of these foods are nutritionally dead. If it comes in a box, can or pouch with a colorful, fancy wrapper, be careful. Read the ingredients.

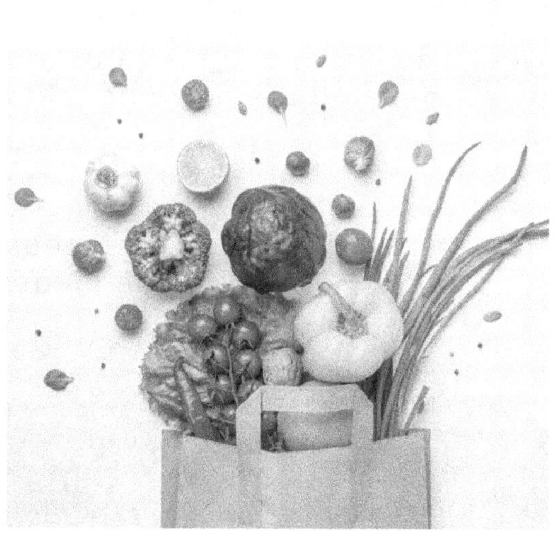

LEVEL 2 FOODS – FRESH/FROZEN FOODS

This would include fresh fruits and vegetables, whole grains, lean organic meats and fish. Whole foods eaten in the form nature made them. When eaten fresh, these foods are full of the minerals, vitamins, nutrients and enzymes your body needs to function properly. Since they are generally low in calories, eating these foods will usually allow you to maintain a healthy weight. These are good food choices to make at your local grocery store or farmers market.

Included in this category would be frozen fruits and veggies as well. Frozen fruits and veggies often retain many of the original nutrients as fresh fruits and veggies but they may lack vital enzymes that are needed for your body to digest them properly. Frozen dinners would be the least nutritious of these foods.

LEVEL 3 FOODS – SUPERFOODS

Superfoods are considered to be a cut above ordinary foods because of their high nutritional value and low fat content, and are concentrated nutrition in small packages. When we speak about Green Superfoods, we are referring to greens that are generally not available at your local store. Not many people go shopping at their local market for Wheatgrass Juice (Powder), Alfalfa, Chlorella, Spirulina, Moringa, Noni, Oat Grass, Barley Grass, Astragalus, and other Green Superfoods covered in this book. In their fresh form, many of the Superfoods cannot be used because they may be bitter, sour, etc. so they may need to be extracted and condensed in order to be utilized by your body.

These green foods are "Super" because they not only contain vitamins, minerals, nutrients, and enzymes to maintain your body, but they also boast an abundance of nutrients that go beyond maintenance and can actually help to support and heal your body.

Green Superfoods have numerous unique phytonutrients, antioxidants and special compounds that can help in the prevention of many illnesses, relieve inflammation and fight conditions associated with aging. Many of these foods only require small amounts be consumed at a time in order to begin deriving the benefits from them. Superfoods not only can supply the nutrients that your body needs to function, they can also begin to reverse health issues that are due to past poor food choices. Scientists have also applied new methods of extracting and concentrating many Superfoods in order to get the most benefit from each of them.

Many of the Superfoods may be unfamiliar to you as they come from exotic places in the world. But these same Superfoods have been used successfully by indigenous people for thousands of years. Much of the research of these Superfoods has been done over the last 50-75 years and has been very encouraging.

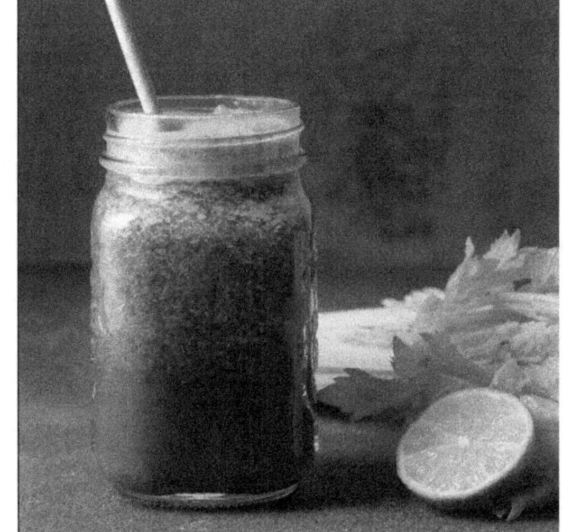

As we do more research, we are finding more and more positive results. You will find much eye-opening research in the references in this book. I encourage you to use the references to do your own research as well.

WHY YOU SHOULD INCORPORATE GREEN SUPERFOODS INTO YOUR DAILY DIET?

Green Superfoods can lower your cholesterol, detox your body, and also protect you from free radical damage, rather like protecting a car from rusting. They are incredibly condensed and highly nutritious foods that offer more health benefits than most other foods. These are the foods that have numerous phytonutrients, antioxidants and special compounds that can help in the prevention of many illnesses, relieve inflammation and fight conditions associated with aging.

Superfoods have superior levels of nutrition, healing properties, and are concentrated nutrition in small packages. Many of these foods only require small amounts be consumed at a time in order to begin deriving the benefit from them. Many are available in the form of dehydrated powders and extracts, which drastically increases the nutrient density. Dehydrated powders are actually more concentrated sources of nutrients than the original Superfoods because the water is taken away. They are also more easily absorbed in your body in this form.

Here are some of the most powerful Superfoods available today :

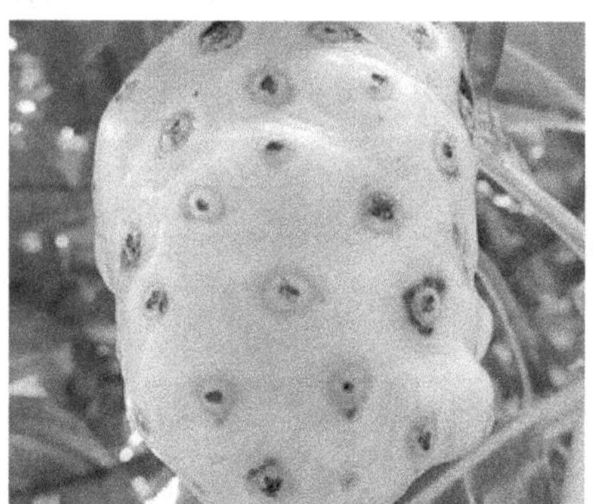

NONI
It is a fruit that has been getting a lot of attention as well, due to its anti-bacterial properties. It also has high levels of anti-inflammatory properties, has been used as a very effective pain reliever, can generate cell repair, and strengthen the immune system. This fruit contains a vast array of vitamins, minerals, phytonutrients, and enzymes. It has also been proven to aid in skin disorders, digestive disorders, headaches, and infections.

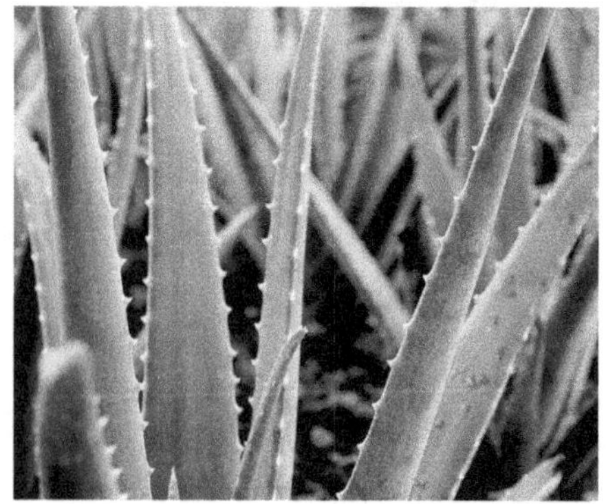

ALOE VERA
Aloe Vera is a very popular super herb thanks to all of its healing compounds including antibiotic agents, amino acids, natural steroids, and an abundance of enzymes and minerals. It is widely used as a skin moisturizer, healer for burns, cuts, acne, bruises, and eczema. It also alkalizes the digestive tract, preventing over acidity which is the common cause of indigestion, acid reflux, ulcers, and heartburn.

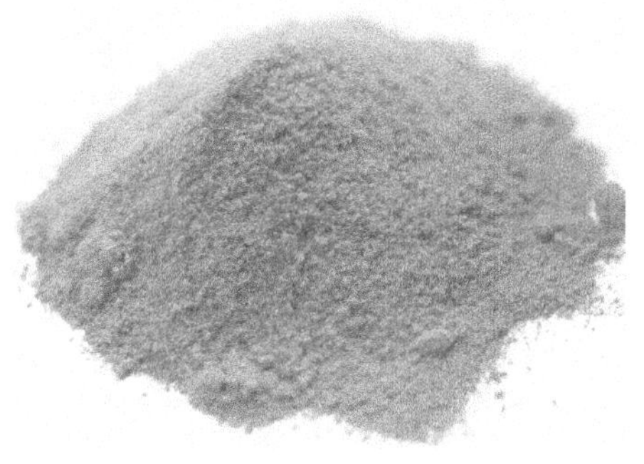

CURCUMIN

Curcumin is the active ingredient that makes turmeric yellow. It is an active compound within turmeric. It is a member of the ginger family and has natural phenols. The turmeric plant is native to India and Indonesia and has been used as a medicine, spice (curry) and yellow dye for thousands of years.

Curcumin provides an anti-inflammatory and cancer preventative component. It is a metabolic regulator as well. Current and encouraging research indicates that it seems to inhibit the growth of certain kinds of tumors, protect against skin diseases, Alzheimer's disease, colitis, stomach ulcers, scabies, diabetes, HIV, uveitis, and viral infections.

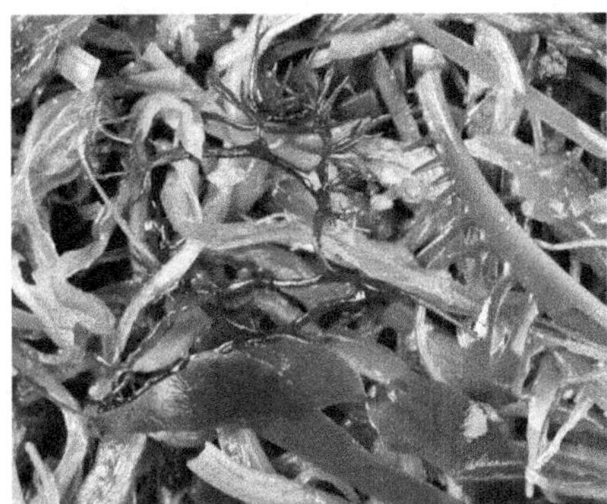

SEAWEED SUPERFOODS

Seaweed Superfoods are the most nutritionally dense plants on the planet and have the most abundant source of minerals within the plant kingdom. Seaweeds are alkalizing and have been shown to help with weight loss due to their naturally high concentration of iodine. This mineral helps to stimulate the thyroid gland, which is responsible for maintaining a healthy metabolism. They are also blood purifying and detoxifying due to their high chlorophyll content, which is a powerful natural detoxifier that draws out waste. Seaweeds also contain antioxidants, which are known for their anti-cancer properties, and offer protection from environmental toxins.

Lastly, seaweed superfoods are amazing in acting as body balancers that help the body actually heal itself! They nourish the entire body when they are consumed, but have the ability to target troublesome areas.

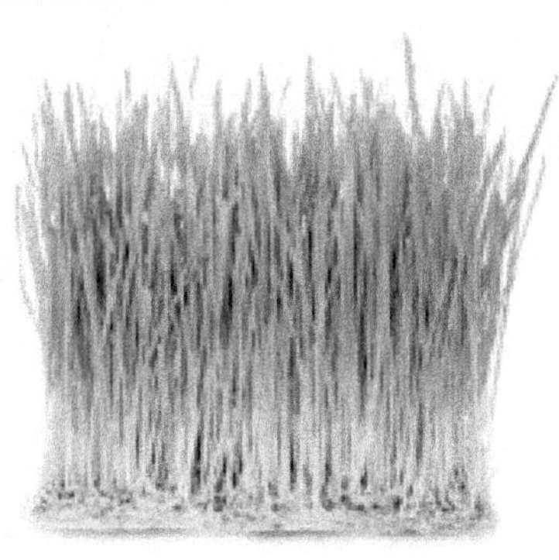

WHEATGRASS

Wheatgrass is an example of a superfood that has been getting a lot of attention recently due to its alkalizing and blood stabilizing effects. It also has the ability to normalize the thyroid gland to stimulate the metabolism, which helps promote healthy digestion, weight loss, and detoxifying effects. It is a sprouted green that does not contain gluten or common allergic agents.

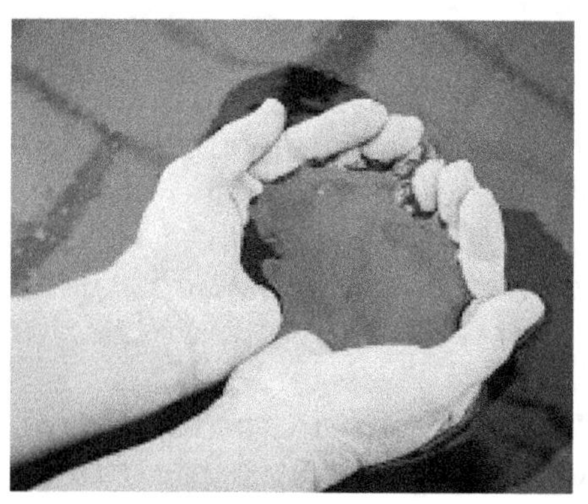

WHITE BLUE GREEN ALGAE
Wild Blue-Green Algae are known as a phyto-plankton and has a 60% protein content and more complete amino acids than either beef or soy beans, as well as one of the highest sources of chlorophyll, beta carotene, and B vitamins. It has been shown to improve memory, brain function, and strengthen the immune system to help with colds, flus, and viruses.

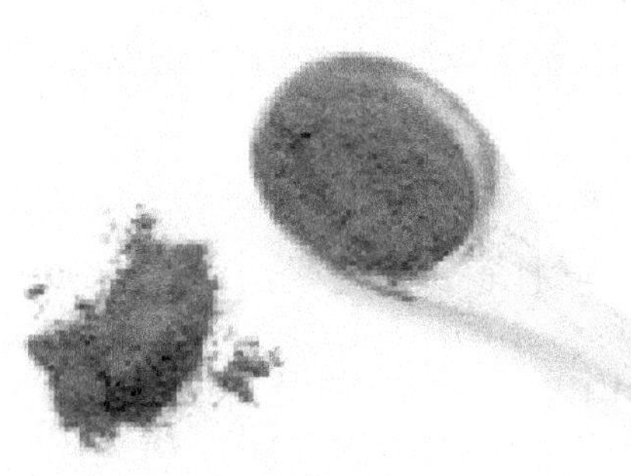

SPIRULINA
Another green superfood is Spirulina, which is a cultivated micro-algae. It is 70% complete protein, beating even steak, which is only 25% complete protein once it is cooked. It has been shown to control blood sugar levels, cravings, assist in weight loss, and has the ability to alkalize your body.

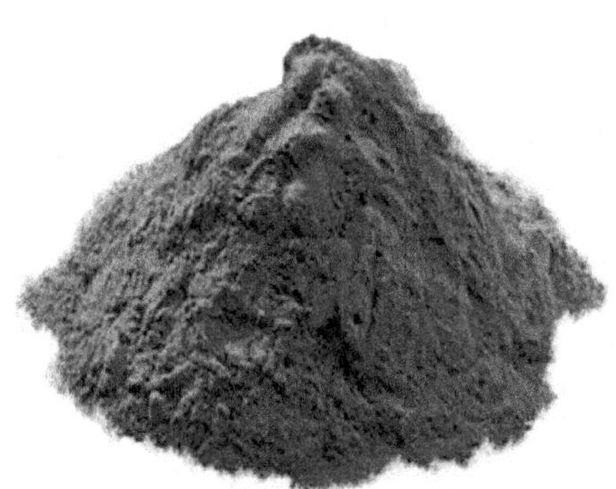

CHLORELLA
Chlorella is one of the oldest and best known living superfood foods on the planet, and grows in fresh water. The nutritional profile of Chlorella provides 50-60% complete protein, 18 amino acids, 20 percent fat, 20 percent carbohydrates, antioxidants such as vitamins C, E, K, beta-carotene, lutein, fiber, chlorophyll, iron, zinc, potassium, phosphorous, biotin, magnesium, calcium, all B vitamins including B-12, Essential fatty acids (EFAs), iodine, iron, and a unique phytonutrient called CGF (chlorella growth factor). Chlorella Growth Factor (CGF) is mostly composed of the nucleic acids, DNA and RNA. Chlorella Growth Factor can help to enhance RNA/DNA functions by providing bio-materials used by your body to rebuild and repair your own DNA and RNA.

HERE ARE 10 SCIENTIFICALLY PROVEN EXTRAORDINARY HEALTH BENEFITS OF CHLORELLA

1. Detoxifies Heavy Metals: Chlorella helps break down heavy metals and toxins such as, DDT, mercury, cadmium, lead, PCB and uranium and keeps them from accumulating in our tissues and organs.

2. Supports a healthy immune system and helps fight infection.

3. Protects the body against ultraviolet radiation. Anyone who has gone through Radiation Therapy and/or Chemotherapy can benefit because Chlorella can help to fight the side effects of those treatments.

4. Chlorella helps fight cancer by strengthening the immune system and improving the action of T cells.

5. Chlorella helps to lower cholesterol, reducing hardening of the arteries, which can be a precursor for heart attacks and strokes

6. Chlorella helps to balance blood glucose levels.

7. Chlorella has anti-obesity effects by reduce cravings, inhibiting the growth of fat cells and helps to normalize the metabolism of fats

8. Chlorella helps with digestion by increasing the good bacteria in the gut, which helps heal diverticulosis, ulcers, constipation, IBS, colitis, and Crohn's disease

9. Helps to enhance RNA/DNA functions responsible for the production of proteins, enzymes and energy at the cellular level.

10. It is the perfect natural multivitamin.

In Japan and China, Chlorella is used as a treatment for: Asthma, colitis, constipation, Cohn's disease, diabetes, diverticulosis, duodenal ulcers, fibromyalgia, gastritis, high blood pressure, high cholesterol, hormone imbalance, hypertension, hypoglycemia, minimizing side effects of cancer radiation treatment, ulcers and ulcerative colitis.

WHAT YOU SHOULD KNOW...
ABOUT CHLOROPHYLL

Green Superfoods are packed with Chlorophyll. Chlorophyll has been the subject of much research lately because of its enormous health benefits.

Here are a few findings.

- Chlorophyll Has **Amazing Oxygen-Carrying Abilities.** It acts like red blood cells in the body; in fact, Chlorophyll has an identical structure to hemoglobin, except that its porphyrin ring centers around a Magnesium atom, not an Iron atom. As a result of this chemical similarity, Chlorophyll acts like red blood cells do, carrying oxygen throughout your body.

- **Wound Healing.** Chlorophyll has long been used as a natural wound healer. It can promote the growth and regrowth of cells, allowing for faster healing. Consuming or using Chlorophyll on wounds can help you heal much more quickly.

- **Cancer Fighting.** Chlorophyll has the ability to fight cancer because of the presence of two chemicals in it, Trisodium Copper Chlorin and Disodium Chlorin. These two chemicals have shown immense promise for fighting cancer cells in animal and human studies. They also tend to dissolve and counteract carcinogens, which are cancer-causing chemicals that we are often exposed to on a daily basis in today's society.

- **Muscle Soreness Relief.** If you are athletic and burn more oxygen than your cells already contain, you get the resulting lactic acid buildup that causes sore muscles. Chlorophyll can actually minimize that by bringing more oxygen to enrich your cells.

- **Anti-inflammatory.** The antioxidants in Chlorophyll are able to reduce swelling and fluid retention, thus easing pain naturally without medications.

- **Antioxidant Action.** Antioxidants fight free radical damage. As a result, they can help reverse some of the effects of aging and degeneration in your body. Chlorophyll is full of a multitude of antioxidants.

- **Alkalizing.** Most bacteria and viruses that attack the human body thrive in acidic environments. You can minimize infection and illness by having a more alkaline body chemistry. Chlorophyll can work to alkalize your body.

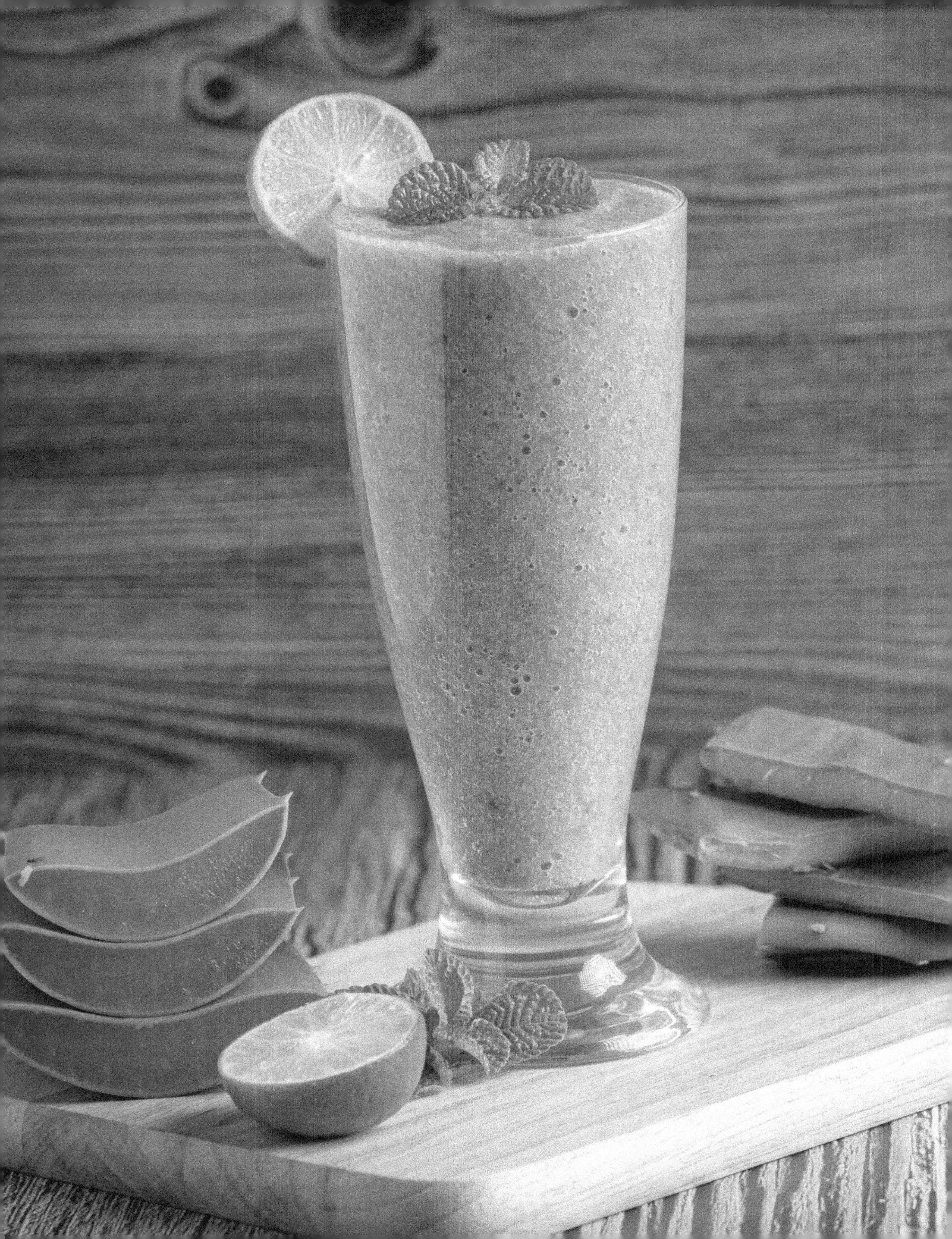

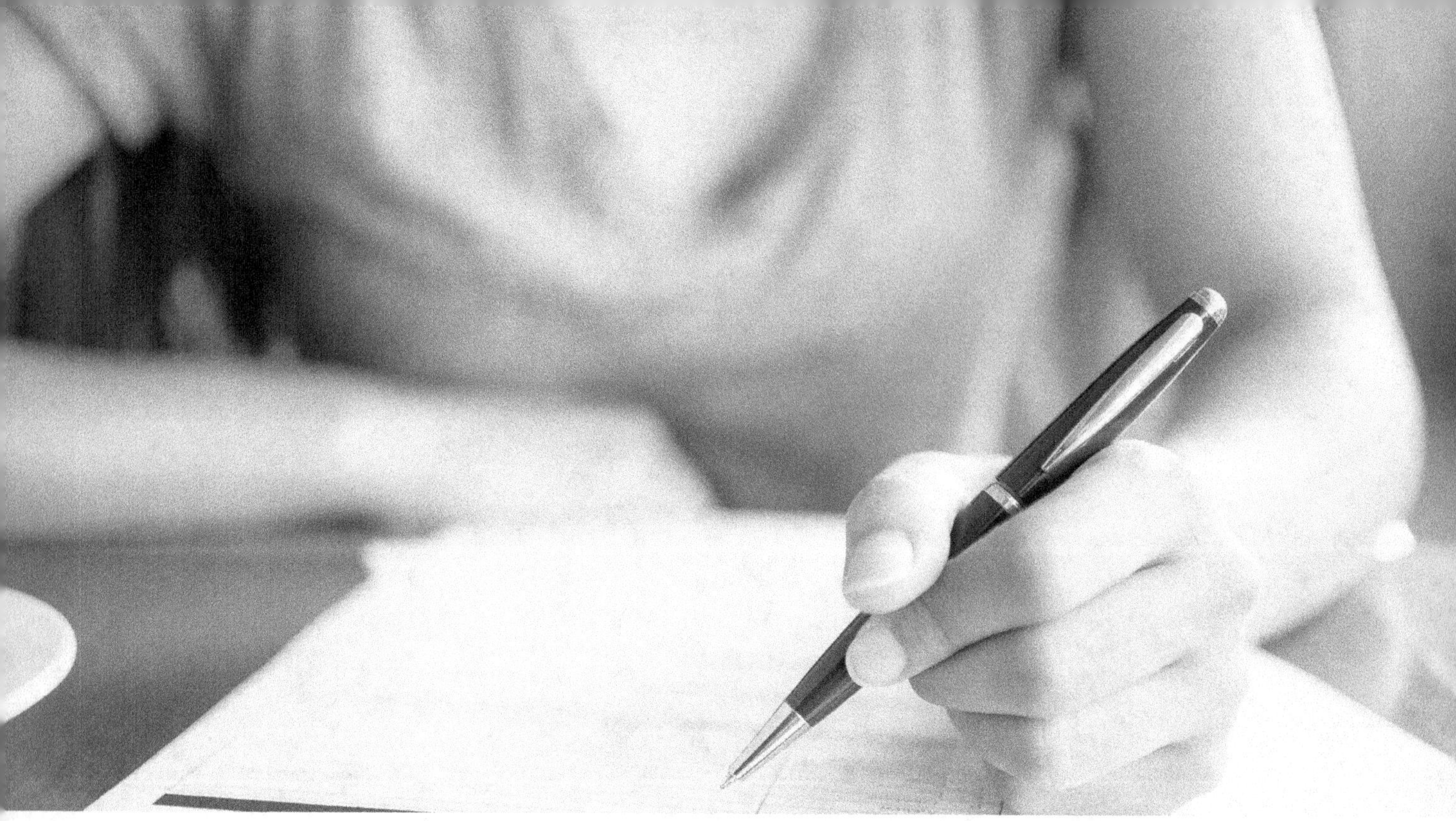

ARE GREEN SUPERFOODS RIGHT FOR YOU? TAKE A QUIZ

- Are you overweight?

- Do you feel sluggish, tired and sick?

- Do you have digestive problems?

- Do you have muscle fatigue and soreness?

- Do you have a desire to cleanse and detox your body?

- Do you want to alkalize your body and balance your pH?

- Do you want to strengthen your immune system?

- Do you want to lose weight?

- Are you vegan or vegetarian?

If you answered "Yes" to any of these, then you are ready to discover the amazing world of Green Superfoods and how they can have a positive impact your health.

- **GREEN SUPERFOODS ALKALIZE YOUR BODY** - If you eat too many acid-forming foods without counterbalancing with alkaline foods, your body struggles to maintain your blood's pH. Normal blood pH needs to be tightly regulated between 7.35 – 7.45. If you eat too many acid-forming foods, it can be catastrophic to your body in many ways. In order to maintain its balance, your body will begin to pull alkalizing minerals out of your bones and teeth, such as Calcium, Magnesium and Potassium, which are essential for proper bone health. Your body will also store excess acid in your muscles, one of the primary causes of fibromyalgia. Green Superfoods are highly alkalizing due to the amount of alkaline minerals they contain (Calcium, Magnesium, Manganese, and Potassium) to name but a few. Also, cancer cannot survive in an alkaline environment and only thrives in an acidic environment. It is good to be alkaline.

- **GREEN SUPERFOODS WILL GIVE YOU AMPLE VITAMINS, MINERALS, AND ELECTROLYTES** in a form that is more easily digestible and readily absorbable than most supplements. All of these Superfoods contain a significant percentage of your daily requirements of each nutrient. Consider Chlorella, which contains 287% of your recommended daily dose of Vitamin A, 71% of your recommended daily dose of Vitamin B2, 33% of your recommended daily dose of Vitamin B3, and 133% your daily dose of Zinc. And that is just one of the Green Superfoods.

- **GREEN SUPERFOODS ARE A SOURCE OF COMPLETE PROTEIN.** You can get a full daily requirement of Protein from these Superfoods, without ever touching meat! For example, Spirulina and Chlorella are a vegan source of complete protein, required for building lean muscle mass.

- **GREEN SUPERFOODS WORK TO SUPPORT YOUR IMMUNE SYSTEM AND HELP YOUR BODY FIGHT DISEASE.** Many of these Superfoods work to strengthen your immune system and help your body fight disease, including cancer. Some of the biggest immune boosters include Spirulina, Chlorella, Lemon, Astragalus, and Noni, as well as others listed in this book.

- **GREEN SUPERFOODS CAN HELP YOU FIGHT OFF RADIATION AND HEAVY METAL TOXICITY.** Many of these Green Superfoods can help you fight off radiation and heavy metal poisoning, which are both serious health issues. Spirulina and Chlorella have shown promise in both arsenic, lead and other heavy metal cleansing.

- **GREEN SUPERFOODS FOR DETOX AND CLEANSE.** Green Superfoods can cleanse your body of impurities and toxins, thus preparing you for serious weight loss and a feeling of well-being. Astragalus is known for cleansing the blood, while Spirulina has shown promise is cleansing people affected by Chernobyl's nuclear radiation contamination. Noni and Chlorella are also often used for their cleansing properties.

- **REGULATE YOUR BOWEL MOVEMENTS AND EASE STOMACH ISSUES.** These Green Superfoods can help regulate your bowel movements and ease stomach issues, such as ulcers or heartburn. Bitter Melon is one of the best sources of natural stomach relief.

- **LOWERING YOUR BLOOD PRESSURE.** Most of these Green Superfoods will assist you in lowering your blood pressure when combined with medical advice from your doctor. Spirulina and Moringa are some of the best sources of natural blood pressure controls and stroke prevention.

- **BALANCING HORMONES, LEADING TO WEIGHT LOSS AND A BETTER MOOD.** Some of these Green Superfoods can also help women balance their hormones, which can help ease pregnancy symptoms, PMS, and mood swings. Oat grass juice is actually one of the best sources of female health relief because of its ability to balance and regulate female hormones, most specifically estrogen.

- **RELIEVE INFLAMMATION:** These Green Superfoods can help you relieve inflammation, which can help ease pain and swelling. Spirulina can ease rhinitis while Alfalfa grass juice minimizes pain caused from swelling joints or sore muscles.

- **HELP FLUSH AWAY CHOLESTEROL.** Green Superfoods will help flush away cholesterol without adding any cholesterol to your diet, helping you defeat high cholesterol readings. Moringa and Noni are great at reducing cholesterol by binding to the cholesterol and helping to dissolve it and flush it out of your system.

For more information about Green Superfoods, see the book, The World's 15 Healthiest Green Superfoods by Maria Tarnev-Wydro, HD.

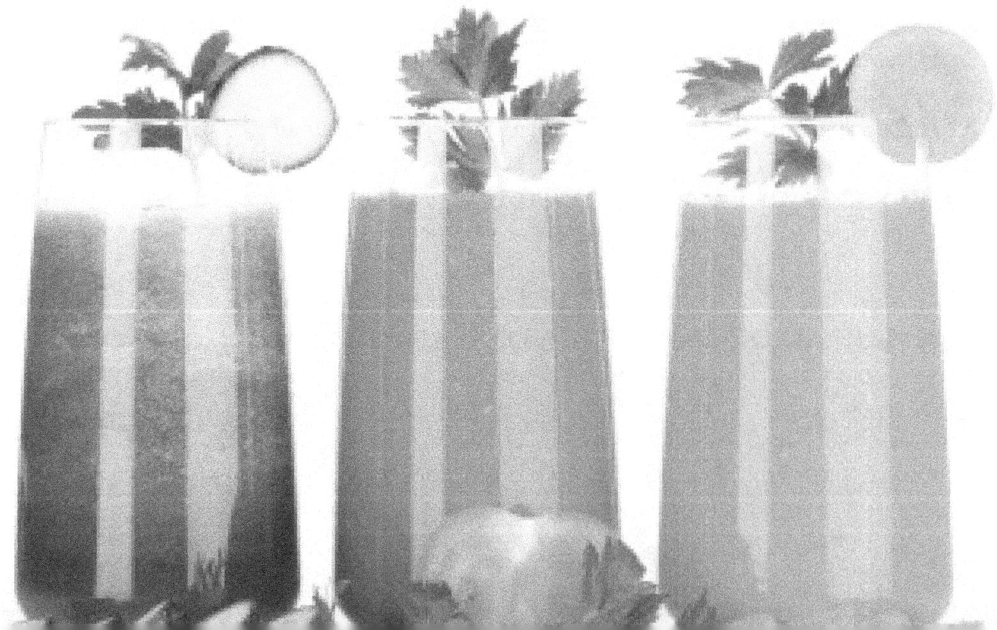

WHAT IS A GREEN SUPERFOOD SMOOTHIE?

It is a delicious nutrient-dense, easily digestible liquid food made by blending leafy green vegetables with superfoods, fruits, fiber and liquid of your choice. Consistency should be like a milkshake and be able to be drawn through a straw.

GREEN SMOOTHIES ACCESSORIES:
You will need the right tools and that includes a quality blender. Vitamix, Breville or NutriBullet Pro are good choices. You will also need Mason jars or storage cups with lids, straws, filtered water, freezer storage bags like Ziploc bags to store veggies and fruits in the refrigerator and/or freezer. You can make your smoothies in the morning and store in the refrigerator to be used all day.

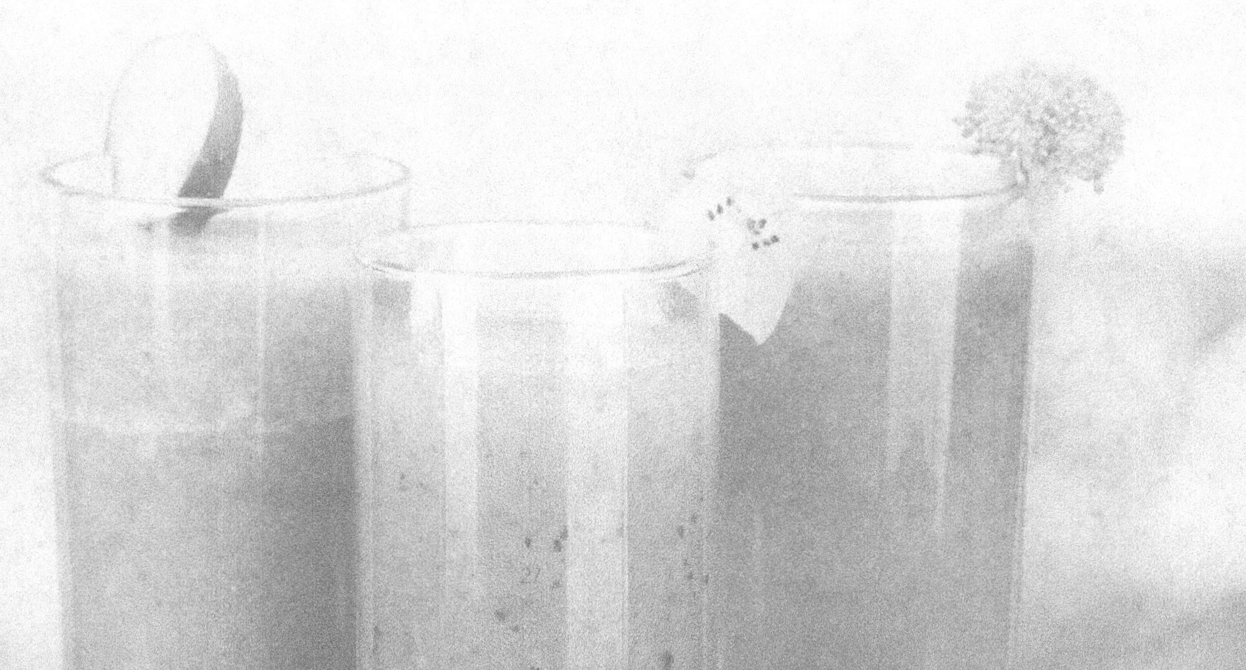

HOW TO CREATE THE PERFECT GREEN SUPERFOOD SMOOTHIE

In order to create your own smoothie from scratch, it is helpful to realize all the different ingredients you can use. Below is a guide to help you *"Mix Your Own"* Smoothie and create your own healthy masterpiece! You can use as many or as few of the ingredients as you want. You can use frozen or fresh fruit, whichever you choose. If you use frozen, decrease ice in the mix.

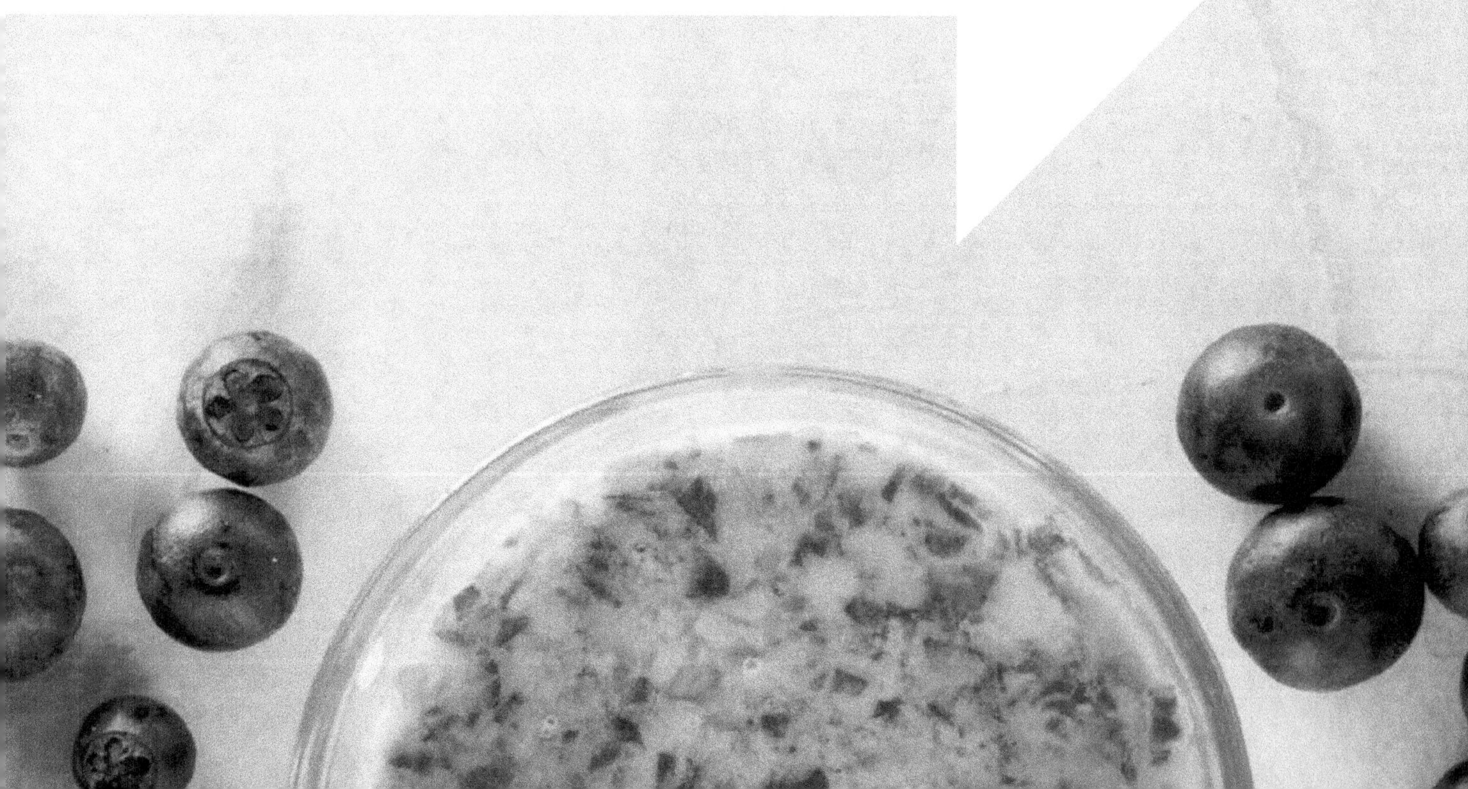

STEP 1. CHOOSE YOUR FRUIT BASE

Peach - Mango
Mango - Banana
Orange - Banana
Pineapple - Peach
Pineapple - Banana
Strawberry - Peach
Blueberry - Banana
Watermelon - Cantaloupe
Strawberry - Banana

Blueberry - Pineapple
Kiwi -Strawberry-Banana
Peaches- Strawberries
Pineapple - Strawberries
Kiwi -Strawberry - Banana
Strawberries - Guava - Bananas
Cranberry - Blueberries - Strawberries
Apple - Blueberries - Bananas

Apple - Strawberries - Bananas
Mixed Berry - Blueberries - Orange
Peaches - Bananas - Mangoes - Oranges
Strawberry - Pineapple - Papaya
Strawberry - Blueberry - Pomegranate
Kiwi – Apple - Orange

STEP 2. CHOOSE YOUR GREENS

Leafy Greens: Mixed Greens, Microgreens, Spinach, Kale, Lettuce, Mustard Greens.
Collard Greens: Swiss chard, Arugula, Purslane, Watercress, Romaine, Dandelion.

STEP 3. FRESH HERBS AND SPICES

Parsley
Mint
Dill
Cilantro
Basil

Turmeric
Ginger
Rose Petals
Lavender
Peppermint

Cucumber
Ginger
Turmeric Root

STEP 4. CHOOSE YOUR SUPERFOODS

Raw Organic Power Shot Greens Superfood Powder from Essona Organics. www.essona.com.

STEP 5. CHOOSE YOUR FIBER

Flax Seeds

Chia Fiber

STEP 6. CHOOSE YOUR LIQUID(S)

Water or Aromatic water
Non diary milk: Almond Milk
Coconut Milk

Flax Milk
Oat Milk
Rice Milk

Hemp Milk
Quinoa Milk
Pea Milk

STEP 7. CHOOSE YOUR EXTRAS

*(All the ingredients below are optional and you can add them
if you wish. Please read the label first).*
Protein Powder: Pea Protein, Chia Protein, Rice, Hemp.
Extracts: Prickly Pear, Berry, Goji Berries, Acai, Hawthorn Berry,
Rose Hips, Maca, Spirulina, Noni, Moringa, Curcumin, Ginseng,
Cordyceps, Medical Mushrooms.
Sweetener: Stevia, Monk Fruit, Yukon Syrup.

PROPER INGREDIENT RATIOS FOR SMOOTHIES

Smoothies are not difficult to make. However, you can gain some insight from the following tips on how to get the most nutrition and the best taste every time. The biggest secret to a good smoothie is following the proper ratio. Otherwise, you might get a liquid mess or something so thick that you can't even swallow it. For perfect, smooth, creamy smoothies that are as appetizing as they are nutritious, follow the ratios below.

With unfrozen fruit, you always want to use 3 parts fruit per 2 parts liquid, 1 part ice. Adding too much ice will make it too thick and impossible to blend, so you should start with 4-5 ice cubes and add more for thicker consistency. Frozen fruit will act as ice cubes, so don't add ice to these. **Try 1 part frozen fruits to 1 part liquid to get the perfect creaminess.** Then add 1-2 tbsp. of your add-in of choice (optional).

Once you have the right ratios, all you have to do is put everything in your blender and turn it on. I suggest a heavy-duty blender with a strong motor and sharp blades. Blend for 30 seconds to 1 minute to make sure all the ingredients are chopped and mixed thoroughly. A large diameter straw makes it easier to drink, especially if it is thick.

It is always best to drink it right away and store any extra in the refrigerator in a Mason jar with the top on.

Pro Tip: If you want to have a more concentrated nutritional smoothie, use frozen fruits instead of ice cubes. You can buy frozen fruits or chop your own and place them in labeled freezer bags. Also, you can use fresh juice in place of water. This will lower the amount of water in your smoothie while keeping the consistency the same. You can freeze any fruits/vegs that are about to go bad. For example, when your bananas are turning brown, peel and chop them and place into freezer bags. Label and place in the freezer. Same with strawberries, blueberries, seedless grapes, mango, and cantaloupe...you get the idea.

IMPORTANCE OF GLYCEMIC INDEX OF FRUITS & VEGETABLES

The Glycemic Index (GI) is a rating system that measures how much a carbohydrate-containing food raises your blood sugar level. The higher the number, the higher the effect on your blood sugar. The standard GI level ranges from 0 to 100. We have included it here for those who need to keep an eye on their GI level and also as a guide to use to balance and adjust your smoothies to your desired range. If you have blood sugar issues, please consult your doctor before preparing any of the smoothie recipes.

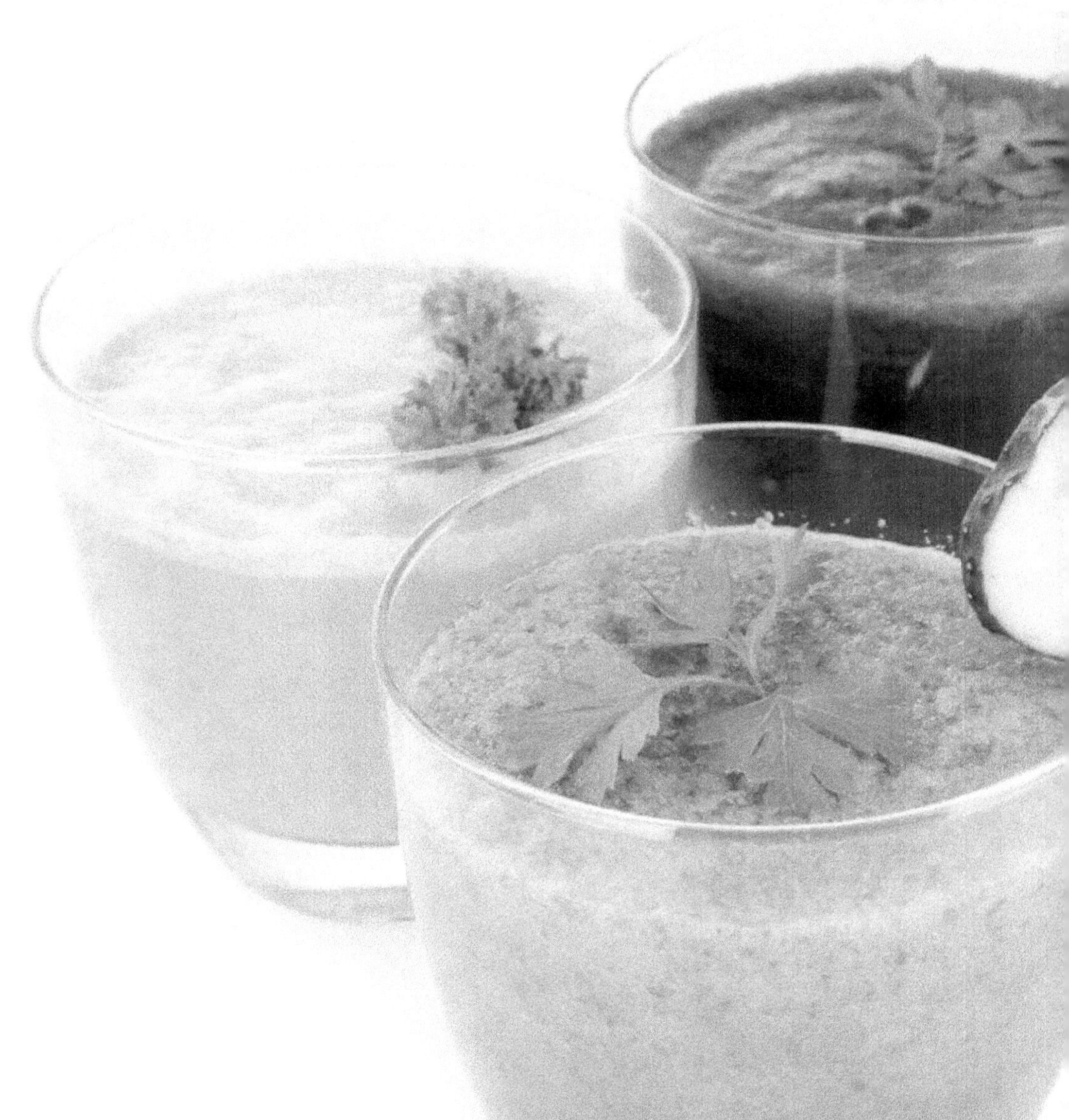

GLYCEMIC INDEX (GI) OF POPULAR FRUITS AND VEGETABLES

FRUITS

Cherries	22	Lime	24	Lemon	25
Peach	28	Nectarines	30	Apple	38
Oranges	44	Kiwi	52	Banana	55
Figs	60	Cantaloupe	67	Guava	78
Apricot	23	Grapefruit	25	Pear	38
Prunes	29	Dates	36	Strawberry	41
Grapes	46	Blueberries	54	Mango	56
Pineapple	66	Watermelon	72		

VEGETABLES

Spinach, Summer Squash, Zucchini, Cucumber,
Green beans, Kale, Lettuce, Dill and Zucchini are 15 (GI)
Collard greens, Beet greens 20 (GI)
Carrots, raw 47 (GI)

INFUSED WATER

To make infused water, start with clean filtered water in a glass pitcher or jar and add your favorite ingredients, allow to infuse overnight. You can then use the water in your smoothies or just mix with Power Shot Greens Superfood blend. Enjoy!

Some suggestions below:

1.   Cucumber, Lime, Strawberry, Mint.
2.   Lime, Ginger Root, Basil.
3.   Watermelon, Honeydew, Mint.
4.   Cucumber, Mint.
5.   Watermelon, Lemon & Lime.
6.   Watermelon & Strawberries.
7.   Orange, Vanilla Bean.
8.   Lemongrass, Lime.
9.   Lavender, Rose Petals.
10.   Cucumber, Lavender

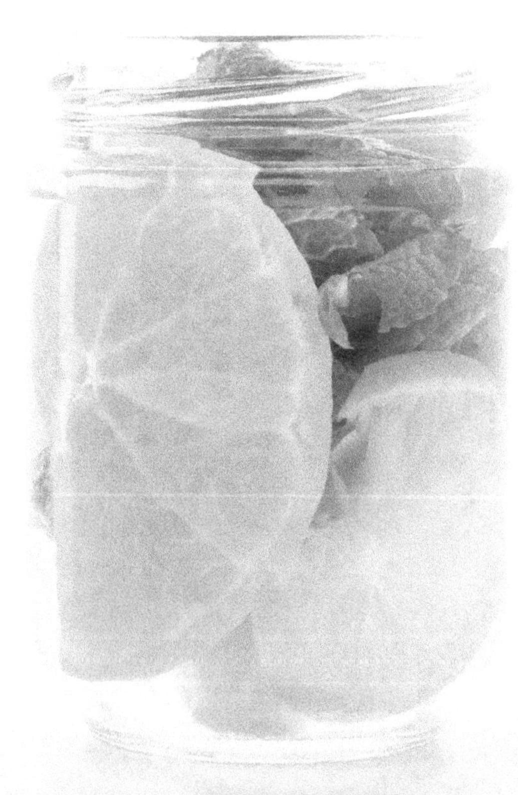

THE 7 DAY GREEN SUPERFOOD SMOOTHIES PROTOCOL EXPLAINED

It is a total of 3 week program with 4 meal plans. Week 1 is a pre-cleanse by slowly and progressively eliminating foods like eggs, dairy, sugar, junk food, coffee, red meat, processed foods, etc. slowly preparing you for the 7 day cleanse. The second week is the 7 day cleanse (follow the strict diet) followed by a 7 day post cleanse to slowly transition you back to a healthy lifestyle. Three weeks total. The only difference is that there are 2 meal plans for week 3. One for vegans and one for flexitarians (includes meat, fish, etc.). Choose the one that is right for you.

For those who are already following a clean food diet, you can start directly with Week 2, the 7 Day Green Superfood Smoothie Cleanse. Each week you have a meal plan, recipes and shopping list. Daily meal plan consists of about 1,200 to 1,500 calories per day. Each meal and smoothies have nutritional info. Each day consists of 3 meals and 2 snacks. You can adjust your calorie intake according to your needs. Each smoothie contains Power Shot Greens Superfood from Essona Organics. It is important to include it because it is an integral part of the entire program.

HERE IS AN OVERVIEW OF THE 3 PHASES

WEEK 1: 7 DAY ELIMINATION "PRE-CLEANSE" PHASE - This is the first stage of cleansing & detoxifying by helping you reduce your toxin load. Take this week to prepare your body. Remove all food obstacles that can hinder your detox and healing.

WEEK 2: 7 DAY GREEN SUPERFOOD SMOOTHIE CLEANSE & DETOX PHASE – This is the actual 7 day detox and cleanse. In this phase, you drink 2 green vegan superfood smoothies daily (one for breakfast and one for lunch) with 1-2 vegan snacks in between and a vegan meal. You can include water and tea as often as you wish.

WEEK 3: 7 DAY TRANSITION "POST-CLEANSE" PHASE - in this phase, you are slowly going to transition back to more solid foods. The Week 3 of 7 Day Transition "Post-Cleanse Protocols" Meal Plans include for Vegan diet (strictly vegan) and Flexitarian diet (includes meat, fish, etc.). You can choose the one that is right for you. In this phase, you drink 1 smoothie daily with 2 snacks in between and enjoy 2 meals. In this transition phase you are focusing on nutrient-dense green superfood smoothies pairing it with delicious whole food meals.

NOTE: *Power Shot Greens Superfood blend from Essona Organics is an integral part of the program. Available at www.essona.com*

HOW TO START

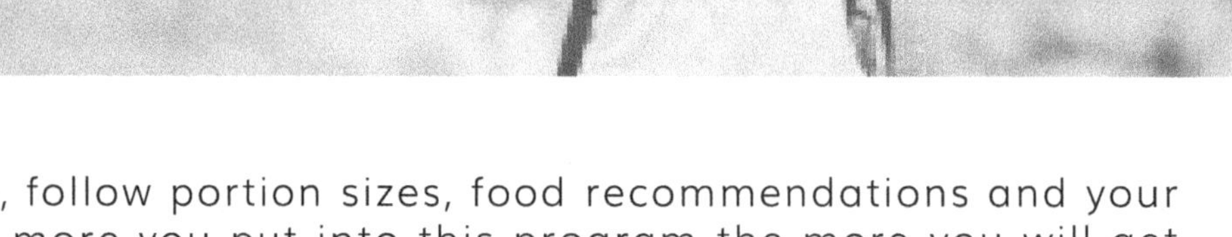

START WITH THE RIGHT ATTITUDE – YOU CAN DO IT!

- Trust the program, follow portion sizes, food recommendations and your exercise plan. The more you put into this program the more you will get out of it!
- Read the entire protocol first to understand the entire process and make preparations ahead of time.
- Before you start this program, consult your healthcare professional (preferably a physician who specializes in integrative medicine) about any medications you may be using. Have them perform a complete physical exam and lab test to determine your present health status.
- As you lose weight and detoxify, your medications may have to be adjusted accordingly.
- Also, before you start your cleanse, it is important to have the following lab tests done to be able to establish an effective, individualized plan for cleansing and healing.

For example, food intolerances can stress your system and give you negative symptoms such as chronic inflammation, weight gain and disease. Ask your doctor to order the recommended lab tests (see below) so you can adjust the meal plans accordingly.

RECOMMENDED LAB TESTS

- Check for allergy, IgG Food Allergy Antibody, IgG and IgE, Allergy Antibody.

- Check for Food Intolerance – Celiac Test (home test) – Biocard Celiac Home Test by 2G Pharma - If you have been suffering from fatigue, diarrhea, vomiting, breathlessness or irritable bowel symptoms, these could be due to Celiac disease. If this is the case, the Biocard Celiac Test may be right for you.

- Check for food sensitivities (blood test) – YorkTest Laboratories has a test you can do online. When I took this test, I found food sensitivities that I didn't expect, like: garlic, eggs, pineapple, cayenne pepper, coconut, vanilla.

Weigh yourself, take measurements of your waist and hips, write it down and take a photo when you start so that you have a record of your starting point. Weigh yourself every morning and keep a daily log.

Set achievable goals - Keep it realistic, it will take longer to lose 50 pounds than to lose 10 pounds. Keep a daily journal of your progress so you can refer back to it when needed. It is best to do the program with a friend (or group) so that you have support (and more fun) together.

Remove temptations by cleaning out your refrigerator and cupboards of any foods that are not on the diet plan and might be tempting to you. Prepare your Shopping List (see List).

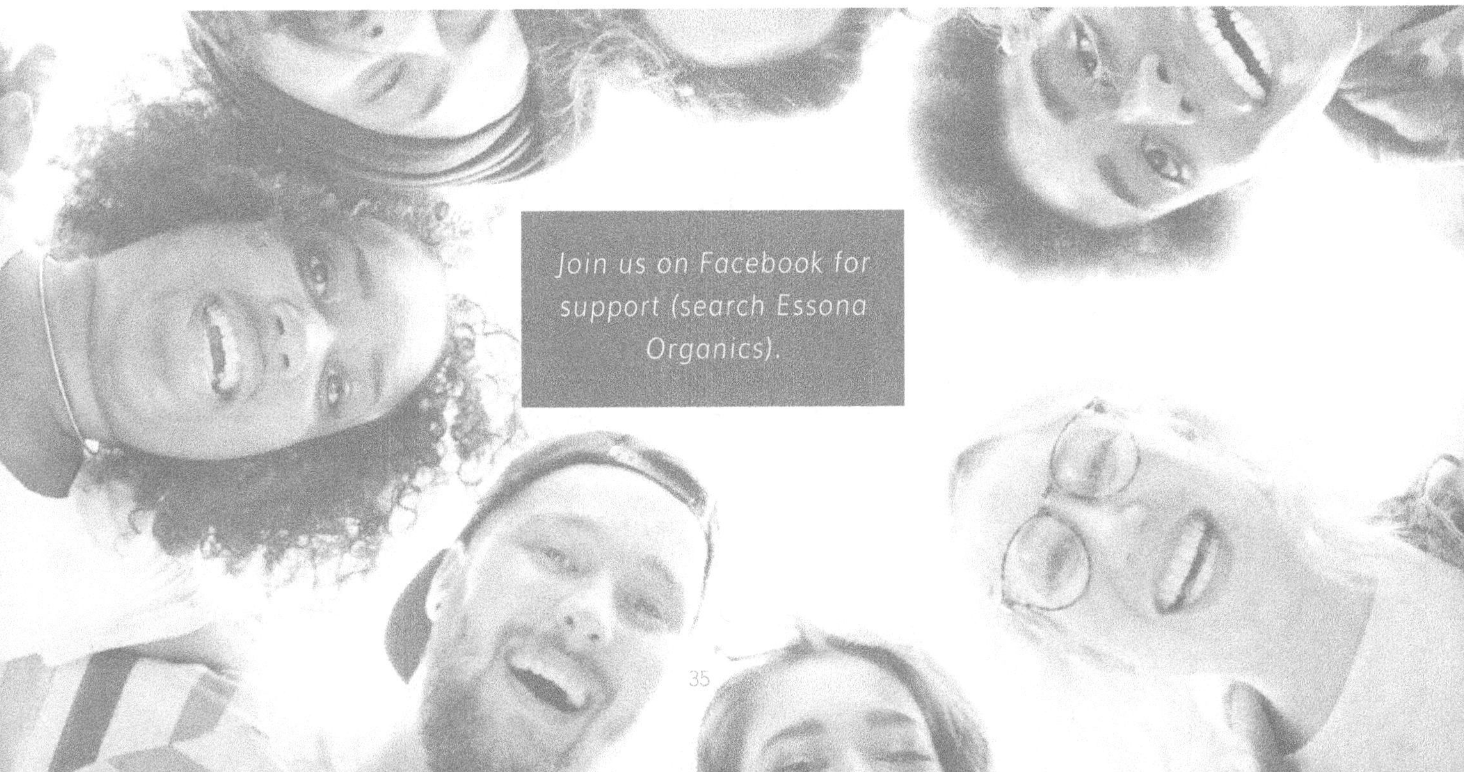

TIPS & SUGGESTIONS BEFORE STARTING

Before you start this program, consult your healthcare professional about any medications you may be using. As you lose weight and detoxify, your medications may have to be adjusted accordingly.

Be sure to schedule your cleanse when you have no special events (weddings, vacation, moving, etc.) For example, December holiday season is not a good choice. January is a great way to start the New Year.

Weigh yourself, write it down and/or take a photo when you start so that you have a record of your starting point.

It is best to do the program with a friend or group so you can support each other (and have more fun!).

Remove any tempting foods from your refrigerator and cupboard.

Make sure to include 30 minutes of daily exercise to allow you lymph system to work efficiently to remove toxins. (Walking, dancing, swimming, biking, etc.).

Start your day with 1 glass (8 oz.) of lemon water. Squeeze ½ lemon into 8 oz. of fresh, filtered water and drink. Allow 15 minutes before eating or drinking anything else.

Buy organic fruit and vegetables if possible. Wash thoroughly.

It is important to rotate different greens with your smoothies. Don't use the same greens every day. Choose from: Romaine lettuce, spinach, kale, Swiss chard, collard greens, turnip greens, etc.

Make sure to sip your smoothies slowly and move it around in your mouth to mix it with saliva to ensure proper digestion. This also allows time to warm the smoothie before you drink it. Drinking it too fast and too cold can cause stomach cramps.

Choose low Glycemic Index (GI) fruits to prevent a spike in your blood sugar. The more sweet juices (sugar) that you drink, the more you will increase your appetite. Combine sweet fruits with bland vegetables to even out the sweetness or you can add some water and sip it a little bit at a time over a 30 minute period.

Do not add any salt, sugar, flavorings or artificial sweeteners to your smoothie.

Leftover smoothies can be frozen as ice cubes to be used instead of ice in the recipe.

Take smoothies and water with you when you leave the house in case you are out longer than expected. Be prepared.

If you have borderline allergies or sensitivities to any fruit or vegetable, please omit it from any recipe. Adjust recipes to your situation and servings needed.

Cooking methods for weeks 1 and 3 include: baking, steaming, grilling, broiling, and boiling. Don't overcook veggies. No frying.

You should take a journal and write down how you feel, if you notice any positives and negatives. Write down any deviations from the original plan.

Once or twice a week, before going to bed you should take a 20-30 minute relaxing bath with baking soda, lavender oil and Epsom salts. The objective is to de-stress and relax your mind, muscles and nervous system. It will also help alkalinize your body and eliminate toxins, improve circulation and sleep quality.

To promote waste discharge and increase toxin removal, you may want to consider a colon cleanse (colonics) and other detox aids during the program.

Take digestive enzymes and probiotics if needed. Especially important for those who have sluggish digestive systems and/or not used to high fiber foods.

Use natural-organic personal care and household items.

REPLENISH YOUR ELECTROLYTES

After sauna, steam, exercise, enema or heavy perspiration you need to replenish your electrolytes. You can do this by drinking 1 cup of coconut water or Homemade Electrolyte Ginger Drink.

Recipe: 4" piece of ginger, peeled, grated, 1/4 cup fresh lemon juice, 2 tablespoons fresh lime juice, peppermint leaves, honey or juice of 1 apple, 1/8 teaspoon fine sea salt, pinch of baking soda, 3 cups coconut or mineral water. To make a ginger juice, grate the ginger, press solids into a fine-mesh sieve, set over a small bowl; discard pulp. Combine all ingredients in a large cup and stir in mineral water. Pour over glass filled with ice. Drink and enjoy!

REST, PLAY AND PRAY

Rest - Researchers have found that people who sleep less than seven hours per night are more likely to develop a variety of health problems and are more prone to be overweight. Lack of sleep can cause imbalances in the hormones ghrelin and leptin that are important in regulation of appetite. Proper rest is a very important to rejuvenate your body, reduce stress, regulate blood pressure and help with proper digestion and nutrient assimilation.

Tips for more restful sleep include going to bed at the same time every night; turning off all lights to make sure your sleeping area is completely dark; getting a foot massage before bed; performing relaxation breathing exercises or prayer before bed and sleeping with an open window (when weather-appropriate) to get clean, fresh air to breathe while you sleep. Also, after eating it is a good idea to take a short rest or "siesta" or "power nap" if possible because your body is using some of its energy for digestion.

Play - It's not just for children. Adults need play time, too. There are many ways for grown-ups to play and have fun: Go to the theater, visit some friends, volunteer at your church, go for a nature walk, exercise, go skiing, running, dancing, rollerblading, or any other physical activity you find fun and enjoyable.

Pray - Having a connection with God has been known to work miracles on health. We have all heard of people overcoming life-threatening illnesses through prayer. Prayer is also a good way to show gratitude for what you have, rather than being bitter about what you don't. As the old axiom says, "I was sad because I had no shoes until I saw a man with no legs." Pray every day and ask for spiritual renewal and guidance.

Let's Get Started!

3 Week
Meal Plans
with
Shopping
Lists

WEEK 1
7 DAY ELIMINATION "PRE-CLEANSE" PHASE

TAKE THIS TIME TO PREPARE YOUR BODY

The first week of the *7 Day Green Superfood Smoothies Cleanse Program* is designed to gradually reduce unhealthy foods and habits to prepare your body for the cleanse. You'll want to begin this one-week prior to your cleanse start date. I cannot stress enough the importance of the "Elimination Pre-Cleanse Phase".

NO MORE..

Processed, boxed, store bought salad dressings, instant food, fast foods and junk food. Refined sugar, processed sweets, baked goods, cookies, alcohol, coffee, store bought juices, soda pop, red meat, pork, cold cuts, cheese, milk, fried foods, hydrogenated oils, soy, corn, aged cheeses, sausages, shellfish.

All foods containing gluten wheat and gluten containing foods (wheat, rye, and barley, bread, pasta, and other products containing refined flour).

Avoid artificial food colors, MSG, additives and preservatives and more.

BECOME A LABEL READER.

You will find a lot of hidden fat, sugar, (corn syrup) salt and other additives in any packaged foods. AVOID THEM!!

DO NOT SKIP THIS PHASE.

In this phase you will be eliminating some foods to prepare for the cleanse.

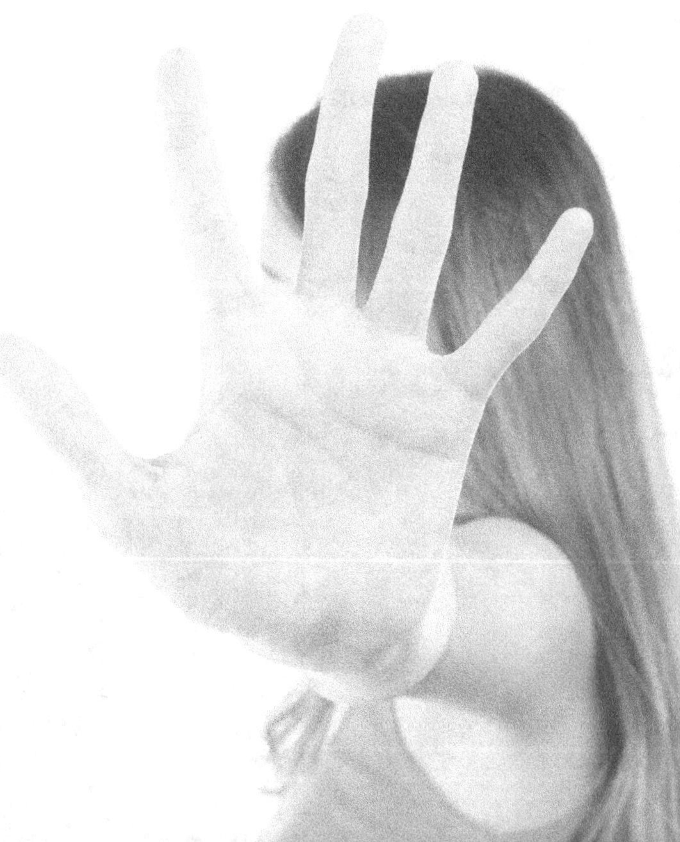

WHAT FOODS TO AVOID?

Avoid foods that are known to cause immediate onset sensitivities such as: eggs, fish, shellfish, nuts, chocolate, peanuts.

Avoid foods causing delayed onset sensitivities: Dairy (casein), chocolate, wheat, soy, corn, & food colorings.

Avoid red meat: Excessive arachidonic acid (from animal fats) stimulates leukotriene production. Leukotrienes are 1,000 times more potent than histamine as a trigger for bronchial constriction and people with allergies. Avoid artificial food colors, MSG, additives and preservatives - especially sulfites which have been linked to asthma episodes, allergy and inflammation (sulfites are common in wine, conventional bottled salad dressings, ketchup, mustard).

Avoid caffeinated products: They contain methyl-xanthines which can increase bronchodilation during asthmatic episodes, stomach upset and heartburn, trouble sleeping (insomnia), headache, nervousness or irritability, rapid heart rate (tachycardia), rapid breathing (tachypnea). Daily use inhibits liver filtering function and can put a strain on adrenals.

Avoid foods containing sulfites: Wine, dried fruit, shrimp, industrial pickles, grapes. Two small glasses of wine are enough to induce a chest oppression and a slight wheezing.

Avoid gluten foods. Gluten refers to the protein of grains capable of aggravating an autoimmune response and may cause problems with your digestive system. Grains containing gluten protein are: whole wheat, wheat bran, barley, rye, triticale, spelt, kamut, couscous, farro, semolina, bulgur, farina, einkorn, durum, wheat germ, cracked wheat, matzo, mir (a cross between wheat and rye).
Processed, grain-based products that may contain gluten are: crackers, bread, breadcrumbs, pasta, seitan, wheat-containing soba noodles, some veggie burgers, cookies, pastries, barley malt, malt vinegar, soy sauce, some salad dressings, sauces or gravies thickened with flour, bouillon and some broths, spice blends, chips.

Avoid refined sugar and refined carbohydrates: Cake, cookies, sweets, crackers, all white flour products, pasta, white rice, doughnuts, refined sweeteners (avoid if possible) white sugar, brown sugar, refined maple syrup, high fructose corn syrup, fructose, glucose, dextrin, dextrose, processed honey, maltodextrin, artificial sweeteners (avoid like the plague!) aspartame, saccharin, mannitol, sorbitol, sucralose.

In short, too much sugar and bad fats, along with a poor diet, can lead to chronic inflammation that can weaken your immune system and is probably responsible for the majority of chronic health problems in America today.

HOW TO PREPARE FOR
7 DAY ELIMINATION "PRE-CLEANSE" PHASE

To prepare yourself for the cleanse, it is important to take 7 days to transition into it. If you already eat a very healthy diet, have a consistent exercise program, don't drink coffee, smoke, eat processed foods, fast foods, meat and etc. it will only take a 4 days to transition smoothly to the cleanse. If you have poor eating habits, give yourself 7 to 10 days to transition. During this phase, you wean yourself incrementally from all dairy products, all meat, and all processed and refined foods

For example, the first 2 days you can eliminate coffee, dairy, sugar, alcohol, processed foods. The next 2 days you can eliminate gluten, red meat, fried foods. The last few days you can eliminate eggs, all meat. The reason for this is that dairy is full of cholesterol and saturated fats, which can lead to artery clogging and plaque formation. Furthermore, animal protein is considered a risk factor for cancer and inflammation. Also, sugar is the root cause of obesity as well as serious conditions such as heart disease, cancer, dementia, type 2 diabetes, depression, acne and infertility. Coffee and alcohol are not allowed in order to improve relaxation and sleep quality. You should take a 30-minute walk every day (or other exercise) to activate your lymph system and help eliminate toxins.

Here is an example of how to slowly
eliminate selected foods throughout Week 1:

DAYS 1-3
What to eliminate: Eliminate all packaged foods, wheat, alcohol, gluten grains, refine sugar, chocolate and alcohol, red meat and peanuts. Avoid dairy & eggs. Start slowly to wean off caffeine.
What to eat: Eat fruits and vegetables in any combination, amount, and preparation using oils and spices as needed.

DAY 3 – 4
What to eliminate: In addition, eliminate any caffeine consumption, this includes coffee, tea, sodas and chocolate. Avoid dairy, grains, nuts and eggs. Also, eliminate all animal proteins.

DAY 5-7
What to eliminate: In addition, eliminate any process foods, vegan or not.
What to eat: Eat only fruits & vegetables in any combination, amount, and preparation using oils and spices as needed. Drink plenty of filtered water.

COOKING METHODS INCLUDE:

- Baking
- Steaming
- Grilling
- Broiling
- Boiling.

Don't overcook veggies. No frying.

The first 4 days you can eat whole plant-based foods with small amount of fresh, organic chicken, turkey and fish. Drinking or using homemade Bone Broth is ok too. Include homemade apple juices, green superfood smoothies, fresh homemade veggie soups, fresh fruits, herbal teas, water (8-10 glasses per day). Eat plenty of raw fruits and vegetables, salads, and non-creamy, grain free soups and add spices and healthy seasonings.

GRADUALLY INCREASING YOUR FIBER

If you're not used to consuming fibrous foods, you want to gradually increase your consumption to get your body used to it. Increasing your fiber too quickly can result in GI issues including gas, bloating and constipation.

DRINK APPLE JUICE & EAT RAW BEET SALAD

As you go through the Meal Plan you may see that there are apples and raw beet salad. The purpose of the apples and raw beet salad is to help thin the bile. Your liver produces bile and sends it to your gallbladder for storage. If your gallbladder is backed up, or the bile is thick and congested, both digestion and liver function can be sluggish. As we want detoxification and elimination pathways functioning optimally, keeping bile flow moving is imperative. Do not consume beet salad with your smoothies. It will create indigestion.

BEWARE OF WITHDRAWAL SYMPTOMS

As you begin to eliminate many of the foods you're used to eating, you may experience withdrawal symptoms. Healing crises commonly occur during a detoxification regimen. Most common symptoms of detoxification include headache, lightheadedness, feeling lousy, diarrhea, cramps, bloating, body aches, fatigue, mood changes, and weakness. These symptoms are due to a combination of factors including: low blood sugar, low fluids, electrolyte imbalance, withdrawal from certain foods and various addicting substances such as alcohol, caffeine, sugar, nicotine. Don't worry, these symptoms will subside as you begin to detox. It may help to drink a cup of ginger or chamomile tea or water. You can also see the Detox Aids section for more suggestions.

KEEP YOUR BOWELS MOVING

Adding a digestive enzyme supplement is also a good idea at this time. It's important to keep digestion optimized and everything moving freely so you can eliminate the toxins as they're liberated. If you're not used to consuming this much fiber, you likely don't have the gut bacteria to break it down adequately. A good enzyme supplement will be helpful here. Your bowels should also be moving daily, ideally, three times per day. If you're not going at least once per day, or it's strained, add a magnesium supplement or drink a small amount of Aloe Vera juice. Increase the amount until you achieve daily bowel movements without strain.

HELPFUL TIPS:

- Address your particular nutritional needs as you go along, such as more frequent snacks, larger meals, and adjusting you calorie intake, increasing protein and healthy fats.
- Take a few minutes each day to do some deep breathing, 30-45 min. of light exercise, positive affirmations, prayer and remember to drink a lot of room temperature water to help flush out toxins.
- Consider 15-30 minutes of sauna or steam room therapy or massage.
- Smoothies and homemade diluted juices should always be taken on an empty stomach and wait at least 30 minutes before eating anything else.
- In the winter, you may substitute frozen fruits for fresh fruits.
- You can add water to any smoothie to thin it if necessary.
- Journaling is encouraged.

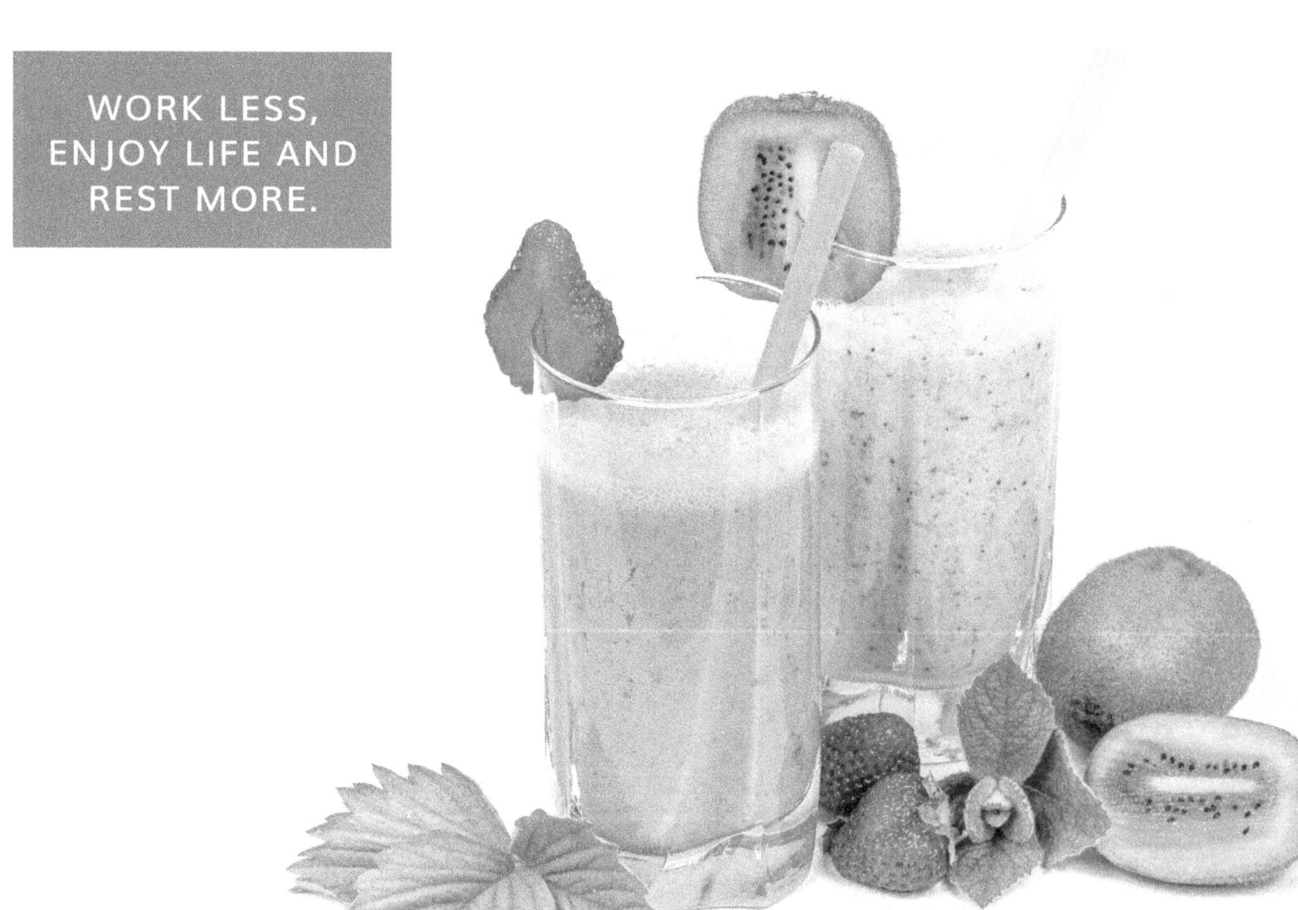

WEEK 1. - 7 DAY ELIMINATION "PRE-CLEANSE" PHASE SHOPPING LIST

FRUITS
Apple 2, medium
Avocado 1 fruit
Banana 3, medium (360 g)
Grapefruit 3, medium
Lemon (juice) 5 fruits
Lime ½
Orange, 1 medium (140 g)
Strawberries (330 g)

SPICES & HERBS
Bay leaf 1
Black Pepper
Basil 2 tbsp.
Chili powder
Cinnamon
Coriander seeds, ground
Cumin
Dill
Oregano, dried
Parsley, chopped 2 cups
Smoked paprika
Thyme, fresh 2 sprigs

CANNED/ PACKAGED ITEMS
1 can diced tomatoes (540 g)
1 can of pinto beans 225 g
Vegetable broth 10 cups
2 cans black beans 1 lb.
Almond milk 315 ml
Coconut Milk Powder 2 tbsp.
Coconut milk, (170 ml)
Coconut or nut butter 1 tsp.
Coconut yogurt, (170 ml)
Hummus 1 tbsp.
Pico de Gallo 60 g
Power Shot Greens
Superfood powder 4 tbsp.
Tofu Extra-firm 90 g
Vegan ground meat ½ -1 cup *(optional)*

FROZEN FOODS
Pineapple, frozen chunks (250 g)
Papaya, frozen chunks (75 g)
Mixed berries (150 g)
Blueberries (150 g)

DRIED FRUIT, NUTS & SEEDS
Chia seeds (15 g)
Dried cranberries 1 tbsp.
Pumpkin seed 1 tsp.
Flaxseeds, 5 tbsp.
Sesame seeds 2 tsp.
Sunflower seeds 14 tbsp.
Walnuts 1 tbsp.,
Chopped almonds, 1 tbsp.

MEAT, FISH, EGG
Meat, Fish, Egg,
Chicken breast, 120 g
Chicken thighs 2 (300 g)
Turkey, ground 210 g

STAPLES
Apple cider vinegar
Extra-virgin olive oil
Flax oil
Italian spice mix
Kosher salt,
Sherry vinegar 2 tsp.
Tamari reduced-sodium
Sesame oil toasted
(dark) Rice vinegar
Vanilla extract

VEGETABLES
Arugula 20 g
Asparagus 6 spears,
Beet, 7 small (560 g)
Bell pepper, 4 large (500 g)
Broccoli (40 g) 1 cup
Eggplant 460 g
Carrots 7 medium
Celery, 4 stalks
Cucumber, 4 small
Cilantro, 6 tbsp.
Cabbage, (70 g) 1 cup
Eggplant 2 slices
Garlic, cloves 10
Ginger 1 tsp, grated
Green beans (220 g)
Kale 10g (1/2 cup)
Leek, 45g (1/2 small)
Lentils 30g
Onion, Red 1¼
Onion, small, 6
Potatoes, small, 5 (700 g)
Peas (60 g) (1/2 cup)
Radishes, 5 (25 g)
Kalamata olives 60 g
Red pepper, roasted 3
Spinach (120 g)
Scallion greens 6, (90 g)
Lettuce leaves 4 large +3 cups
Tomato, 5 medium (550 g)
Zucchini, 2 medium
Swiss chards (36 g) 1 cup
Shallot, 1 small

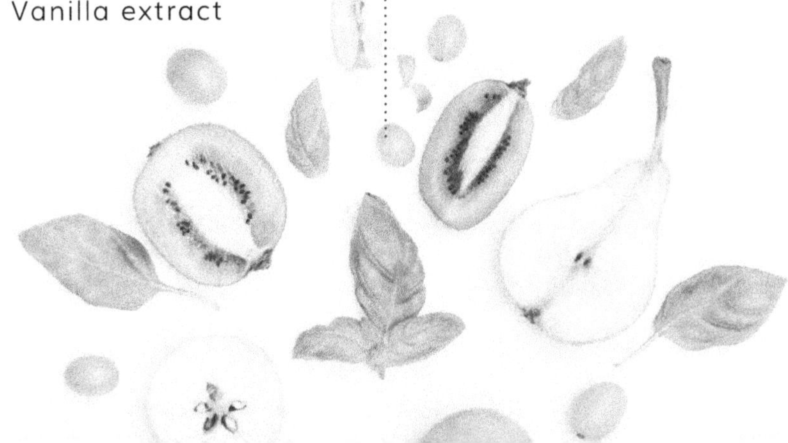

WEEK 1. - 7 DAY ELIMINATION "PRE-CLEANSE" PHASE WEEKLY MEAL PLAN

	DAY 1	DAY 2	DAY 3	DAY 4	DAY 5	DAY 6	DAY 7
I MEAL	1 cup Lemon-Ginger drink or Water or Detox tea	1 cup Lemon-Ginger drink or Water or Detox tea	1 cup Lemon-Ginger drink or Water or Detox tea	1 cup Lemon-Ginger drink or Water or Detox tea	1 cup Lemon-Ginger drink or Water or Detox tea	1 cup Lemon-Ginger drink or Water or Detox tea	1 cup Lemon-Ginger drink or Water or Detox tea
	1 serving Green Enzyme Smoothie	1 serving Banana Cinnamon Oatmeal	1 serving Coconut Yogurt Berry Bowl	1 serving Green Banana Coconut Smoothie	1 serving Coconut Yogurt with Bananas and Chia Seeds	1 serving Coconut Yogurt Berry Bowl	1 serving Green Strawberry Smoothie
SNACK	1 oz. Pumpkin seeds or mixed seeds	1 Grapefruit	1 Apple	1 Grapefruit	10 carrot sticks + 2 tbsp. of seed butter	1 Grapefruit	1 Apple
II MEAL	1 cup Detox Tea/Water	1 cup Detox Tea/Water	1 cup Detox Tea/Water	1 cup Detox Tea/Water	1 cup Detox Tea/Water	1 cup Detox Tea/Water	1 cup Detox Tea/Water
	1 serving Mediterranean Grilled Veggie Wrap	1 serving Turkey Meatball Veggie Soup w/Green Salad	1 serving Lettuce Taco Chicken Wrap	1serving Lemon Chicken Soup with Greek Salad	1 serving Hawaiian Poke Bowl	1 serving of Rice Tortilla Wrap with veggies	1 serving Green Bean Stew
SNACK	Raw Beet Salad with seeds	½ serving Raw Beet Salad with seeds	½ serving Raw Beet Salad with seeds	Raw Beet Salad with seeds	½ serving Raw Beet Salad with seeds	Raw Beet Salad with seeds	Raw Beet Salad with seeds
III MEAL	1 cup Detox Tea/Water	1 cup Detox Tea/Water	1 cup Detox Tea/Water	1 cup Detox Tea/Water	1 cup Detox Tea/Water	1 cup Detox Tea/Water	1 cup Detox Tea/Water
	1 serving Turkey Meatball Veggie Soup w/ /Grilled Veggies	1 serving Stuffed Bell Pepper w/ ground turkey	1 serving Lemon Chicken Soup with Green Salad	1 serving Vegan Chili	1 serving of Lentil Soup with Greens with Grilled Veggies Salad	1 serving of Lentil Soup with Greens with Greek Salad	1 serving Cranberry Cilantro Quinoa Salad
	whole day kcal	whole day kcal	whole day kcal	whole day kcal	whole day kcal	whole day kcal	whole day kcal
	1226	1451	1497	1467	1424	1272	1394

WEEKLY AVERAGE 1390 KCAL PER DAY

WEEK 1. - 7 DAY ELIMINATION "PRE-CLEANSE" PHASE DAILY MEAL PLAN

DAY 1

	1 cup of Lemon-Ginger /Water
Breakfast:	Green Enzyme Smoothie
	1 cup detox tea/ distilled water
Snack 1:	1 oz. of pumpkin or mixed roasted seeds
Lunch:	Mediterranean Grilled Veggie Wrap
	2 cup detox tea/water
Snack 2:	Raw Beet Salad with seeds
Dinner:	Turkey Meatball Veggie Soup with Grilled Veggies

DAY 2

	1 cup of Lemon-Ginger /water
Breakfast:	Banana Cinnamon Oatmeal
	1 cup detox tea/water
Snack 1:	Grapefruit (260g)
Lunch:	Turkey Meatball Veggie Soup with Green Salad
	2 cup detox tea/water
Snack 2:	Raw Beet Salad with seeds (½ serving)
Dinner:	Stuffed Bell Peppers with Ground Turkey
	2 cup detox tea/water

DAY 3

	1 cup of Lemon-Ginger water
Breakfast:	Coconut Yogurt Berry Bowl
	1 cup detox tea/water
Snack 1:	1 Apple (180g)
Lunch:	Lettuce Taco Chicken Wrap
	2 cup detox tea/water
Snack 2:	Raw Beet Salad with seeds (½ serving)
Dinner:	Lemon Chicken Soup with Green Salad
	2 cup detox tea/water

DAY 4

	1 cup of Lemon-Ginger /Water
Breakfast:	Green Banana Coconut Smoothie
	1 cup detox tea/water
Snack 1:	1 Grapefruit
Lunch:	Lemon Chicken Soup with Greek Salad
	1 cup detox tea/water
Snack 2:	Raw Beet Salad with seeds
Dinner:	Vegan Chili
	2 cup detox tea/water

DAY 5

	1 cup of Lemon-Ginger /water
Breakfast:	Coconut Yogurt w/Banana & Chia Seeds Bowl
	1 cup detox tea/water
Snack 1:	10 carrot sticks (80g) with 2 tbsp. of Tahini spread
Lunch:	Hawaiian Poke Bowl
	1 cup detox tea/water
Snack 2:	½ serving Raw Beet Salad with seeds (½ serving)
Dinner:	Lentil Soup with Grilled Veggies Salad

DAY 6

	1 cup of Lemon-Ginger water
Breakfast:	Coconut Yogurt Berry Bowl
	1 cup detox tea/water
Snack 1:	1 Grapefruit (260g)
Lunch:	Rice Tortilla Wrap with Veggies
	1 cup detox tea/water
Snack 2:	Raw Beet Salad with seeds
Dinner:	Lentil Soup with Greek Salad
	1 cup detox tea/water

DAY 7

	1 cup of Lemon-Ginger water
Breakfast:	Green Strawberry Smoothie
	1 cup detox tea/water
Snack 1:	1 Apple (180g)
Lunch:	Green Bean Stew
	1 cup detox tea/water
Snack 2:	Raw Beet Salad with seeds
Dinner:	Cranberry Cilantro Quinoa Salad
	1 cup detox tea/water

WEEK 2
7 DAY GREEN SUPERFOOD SMOOTHIE "CLEANSE & DETOX" PHASE

Welcome to Week 2 of the **7 Day Green Superfood Smoothies Cleanse.** This is the cleanse and detox week. There is no meat or dairy or eggs allowed in this week. You will be eating primarily fresh fruits and vegetables with small amounts of seeds and nuts (omit nuts if you are allergic). The smoothies you will be making are made from organic fruits and vegetables and are full of valuable enzymes that will provide your body with additional energy. If the juice tastes too strong, you can dilute it with water.

The aim of this week is to flood your body with super nutrition while allowing it to cleanse and detoxify. You will also notice that you will begin losing weight and your energy level will increase. You may also notice that you are sleeping better.

WHAT TO EAT

Each day you drink 2 fresh homemade Green Superfood Smoothies (from your blender at home, not store-bought), 16 ounces each for breakfast and lunch, and eat one homemade healthy soup for dinner. There are 2 snacks between meals along with water and Detox Tea. Each daily meal plan is about 1,200-1,400 calories per day. You can snack on celery, carrots, cauliflower, cucumbers, apples, avocado, grapefruit anytime you are hungry. Also, on day 1-4 you can use handful of unsalted seeds like pumpkin seeds, sunflower seeds, chia seeds, flax seeds, walnuts or almonds (no nuts if you are allergic to nuts).

· FOLLOW THE PLAN.

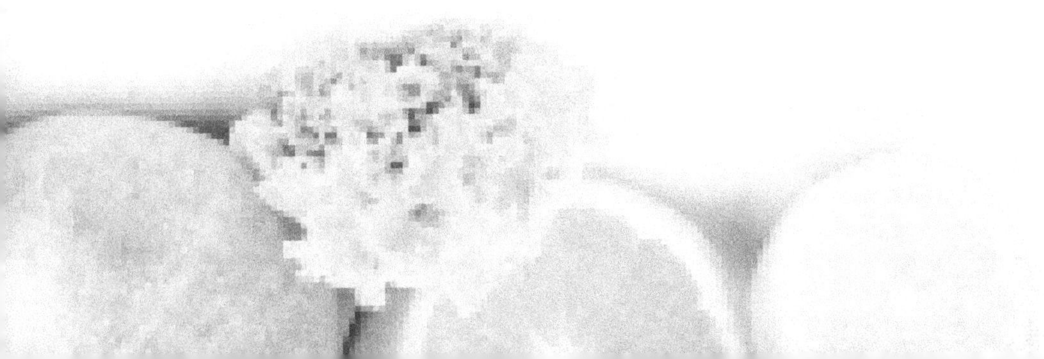

HERE IS A SAMPLE DAILY SCHEDULE BELOW:

Morning:	lemon water + smoothie + detox tea + snack-water
Lunch:	smoothie + detox tea+ snack-water
Dinner:	soup + detox tea or water
Detox aids:	Supplements (optional).

If you would like to incorporate Intermittent Fasting, skip breakfast smoothie.

HELPFUL TIPS:

- You can pre-make your smoothies for the whole day (32-40 oz.). Keep refrigerated.
- Just before you drink the smoothies add your Power Shot Greens Superfood Blend.
- Also, consider using a sauna daily if you have access to one. The sweating produced by a sauna will help to increase elimination through your pores. Be sure to always rinse off with cool water after sauna use to wash away the released toxins.

REMEMBER TO DRINK WATER AND EXERCISE DAILY.

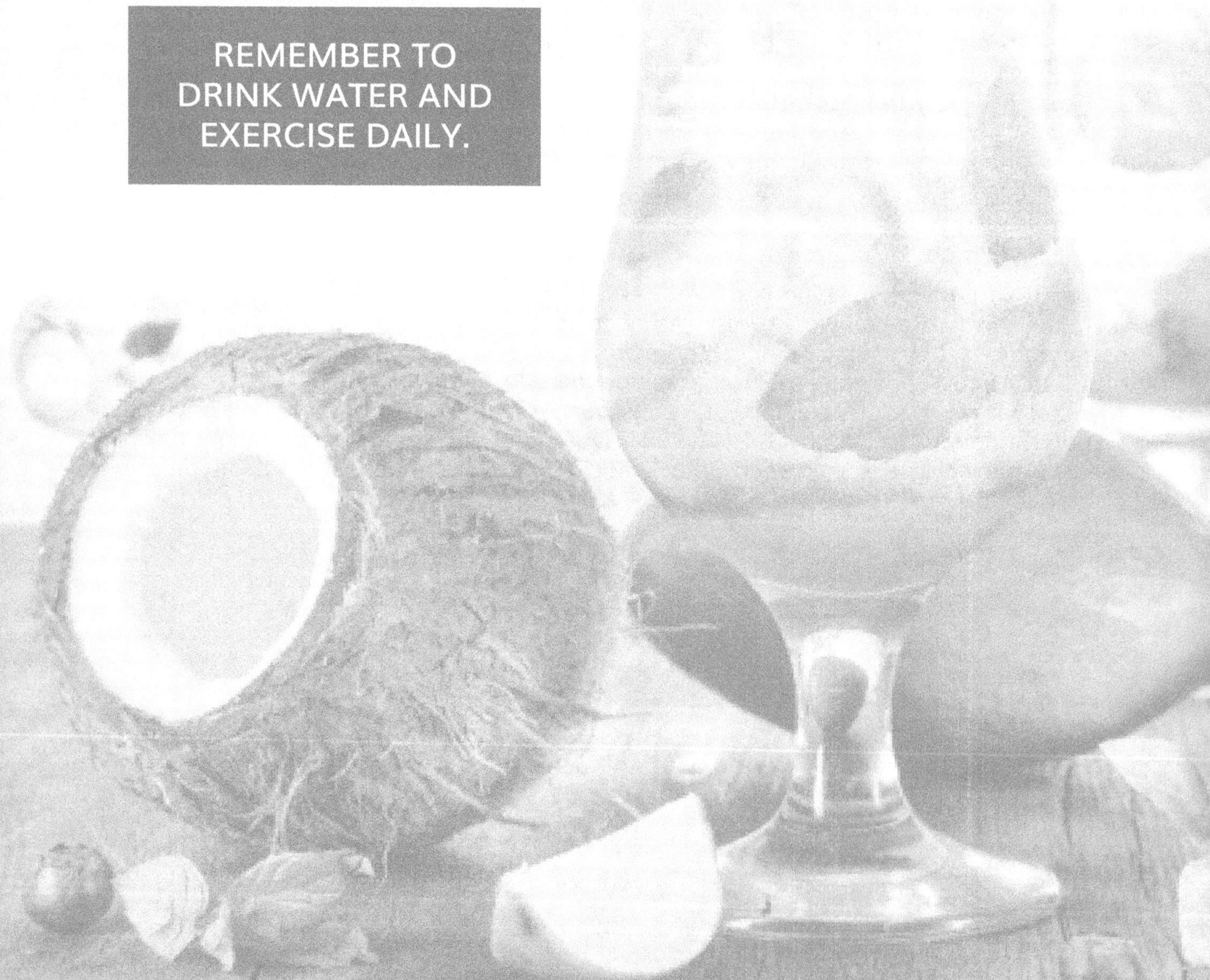

WEEK 2. 7 DAY GREEN SUPERFOOD SMOOTHIE "CLEANSE & DETOX" PHASE SHOPPING LIST

FRUITS
Apple 2 large (440 g)
or 1 lb.
Apple, 7 medium
(1260 g) or 2.8lb
Avocado, 2.5 (400 g)
Grapefruit 5 large
(1650 g) or 3.6 lb.
Grapes, seedless
80 g or 2.8oz
Melon chunks 160 g
or 5.3 oz.
Lemon, 2 fruit

SPICES & HERBS
Mint
Black pepper
Oregano
Basil
Bay leaves
Cayenne pepper
Garlic powder

CANNED/ PACKAGED ITEMS
Coconut milk ½ cup
Coconut milk powder 1
tbsp. veggie broth 14 cups
vegetable Juice V8, 1 cup
Crispy tofu cubes 5 oz.
Coconut yogurt 1 ½ cup
 Power Shot Greens
Superfood powder 7 tbsp.
Peppermint tea
Tahini-Lemon spread 14
tbsp. or (210 g) or 7 oz.

FROZEN FOODS
Blueberries (140 g)
Mixed berries (440 g)
Pineapple chunks,
(440 g)
mango-peach mix
(300 g)
honeydew chunks,
1 cup

DRIED FRUIT, NUTS & SEEDS
Pumpkin or mixed seeds
(150 g) or 5 oz.
Sunflower seeds (30 g)
or 1 oz.
flaxseed, ground
12 tbsp.
Chia seeds (180 g)
or 6 oz.
Cashews 1 tbsp.

STAPLES
Apple cider vinegar
Kosher salt,
Sunflower or
grape seed oil

GRAINS & PRODUCTS
Rice short Grain (100g)

VEGETABLES
Bell pepper, 1
Bok Choy (420 g)
or 14 oz.
Broccoli 1 cup (40 g)
Cabbage, (620 g)
or 1.4 lb.
Carrot 6 medium (420
g) or 14 oz.
Cauliflower (110 g)
or 4 oz.
Cucumber (500 g) ~
3 smaller
Celery 3 stalk (120 g)
or 4 oz. Garlic,
10 cloves
Greens mixed (30 g)
or 1 oz.
Ginger root, 1 small
Spinach, (330 g) or 11
oz.
Scallions, 8 large
Shiitake mushrooms
dried 7~ (125 g)
Kale (90 g) or 3 oz.
Onions, 5 medium sized
Leeks, 4 small
Lettuce 3 cups
Potatoes (450 g) or 1 lb.
Tomatoes, 8 medium
Parsley, fresh 1 ½ tbsp.

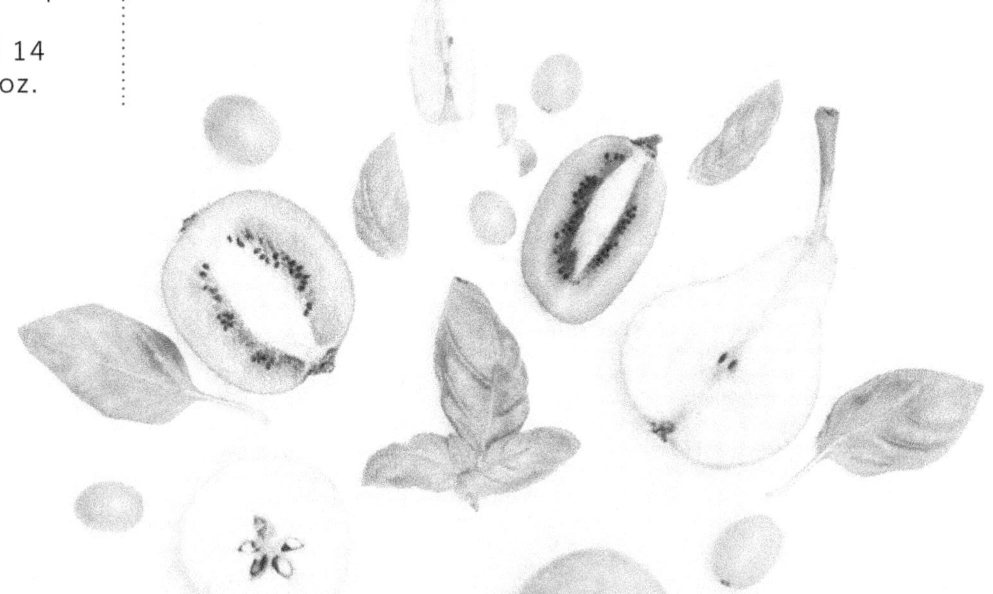

WEEK 2: 7 DAY GREEN SUPERFOOD SMOOTHIE "CLEANSE & DETOX" PHASE WEEKLY MEAL PLAN

	DAY 1	DAY 2	DAY 3	DAY 4	DAY 5	DAY 6	DAY 7
I MEAL	1 cup Lemon-Ginger drink or Water or Detox tea	1 cup Lemon-Ginger drink or Water or Detox tea	1 cup Lemon-Ginger drink or Water or Detox tea	1 cup Lemon-Ginger drink or Water or Detox tea	1 cup Lemon-Ginger drink or Water or Detox tea	1 cup Lemon-Ginger drink or Water or Detox tea	1 cup Lemon-Ginger drink or Water or Detox tea
	1 serving of Green Apple Berry Smoothie	1 serving Green Pina Colada Smoothie	1 serving of Green Mango Peach smoothie	1 serving of Green Strawberry Smoothie	1 serving Green Melon Smoothie	1 serving Green Honeydew Smoothie	1 serving Green Green Mango Kale Smoothie
SNACK	10 celery sticks + 2 tbsp. Tahini-Lemon spread	1 Avocado, sliced	1 cup of Sliced Strawberries + 2 tbsp. Of Tahini Spread	60g of Sunflower Seeds	1 Apple, large	10 Carrot Sticks + 2 tbsp. of Tahini Spread	1 oz. Pumpkin seeds or mix seeds
II MEAL	1 cup Lemon-Ginger drink or Water or Detox tea	1 cup Lemon-Ginger drink or Water or Detox tea	1 cup Lemon-Ginger drink or Water or Detox tea	1 cup Lemon-Ginger drink or Water or Detox tea	1 cup Lemon-Ginger drink or Water or Detox tea	1 cup Lemon-Ginger drink or Water or Detox tea	1 cup Lemon-Ginger drink or Water or Detox tea
	1 serving of Green Apple & Berry Smoothie	1 serving Green Pina Colada Smoothie	1 serving of Green Mango Peach Smoothie	1 serving of Green Strawberry Smoothie	1 serving Green Melon Smoothie	1 serving Green Honeydew Smoothie	1 serving of Green Mango Kale Smoothie
SNACK	Raw Beet Salad with seeds	½ serving Raw Beet Salad with seeds	½ serving Raw Beet Salad with seeds	Raw Beet Salad with seeds	½ serving Raw Beet Salad with seeds	Raw Beet Salad with seeds	Raw Beet Salad with seeds
III MEAL	1 cup Detox Tea/Water	1 cup Detox Tea/Water	1 cup Detox Tea/Water	1 cup Detox Tea/Water	1 cup Detox Tea/Water	1 cup Detox Tea/Water	1 cup Detox Tea/Water
	1 serving Cabbage Detox Soup 1 large grapefruit	1 serving Cabbage Detox Soup	1 serving of Green Power Soup, 10 carrot sticks + 2 tbsp. of tahini spread	1 serving of Green Power Soup , 1 large grapefruit	1 serving Hippocrates Healing Soup, 1 large grapefruit	1 serving Hippocrates Healing Soup, 1 medium apple	Seaweed Congee Chinese Rice Porridge with Cucumber Dill Salad
	whole day kcal	whole day kcal	whole day kcal	whole day kcal	whole day kcal	whole day kcal	whole day kcal
	1213	1541	1312	1267	1147	1267	1441

WEEKLY AVERAGE 1311 KCAL PER DAY

WEEK 2: 7 DAY GREEN SUPERFOOD SMOOTHIE "CLEANSE & DETOX" PHASE WEEKLY MEAL PLAN

DAY 1

	1 cup of Lemon-Ginger /Water
Breakfast:	Green Apple Berry Smoothie
	1 cup detox tea/water
Snack 1:	10 celery sticks cut into strips (40 g) +
	2 tbsp. of Tahini-Lemon spread (14 g)
Lunch:	Green Apple Berry Smoothie
	1 cup detox tea/water
Snack 2:	30g or 2 oz. of pumpkin or mixed seeds
Dinner:	Cabbage Detox Soup
	1 cup detox tea/water
	1 large grapefruit

DAY 2

	1 cup of Lemon-Ginger /water
Breakfast:	Green Pina Colada Smoothie
	1 cup detox tea/water
Snack 1:	Avocado, sliced (200 g)
Lunch:	Green Pina Colada Smoothie
	1 cup detox tea/water
Snack 2:	1 Apple, medium (180 g)
Dinner:	Cabbage Detox Soup
	1 cup detox tea/water

DAY 3

	1 cup of Lemon-Ginger water
Breakfast:	Green Mango Peach Smoothie
	1 cup detox tea/water
Snack 1:	1 cup of strawberries (145 g) +
	2 tbsp. of Tahini spread (14 g)
Lunch:	Green Mango Peach Smoothie
	1 cup detox tea/water
Snack 2:	Half of a cucumber (100 g cut into sticks) +
	avocado dip (100 g)
Dinner:	Green Power Soup
	1 cup detox tea/water
	10 carrot sticks (70 g) + 2 tbsp. of tahini spread

DAY 4

	1 cup of Lemon-Ginger /Water
Breakfast:	Green Strawberry Smoothie
	1 cup detox tea/water
Snack 1:	60g of Sunflower Seeds
Lunch:	Green Strawberry Smoothie
	1 cup detox tea/water
Snack 2:	1 Apple, large (220 g) + 3 tbsp. of Tahini spread (45 g)
Dinner:	Green Power Soup
	1 cup detox tea/water
	1 large grapefruit

DAY 5

	1 cup of Lemon-Ginger /water
Breakfast:	Green Melon Smoothie
	1 cup detox tea/water
Snack 1:	1 Apple
Lunch:	Green Melon Smoothie
	1 cup detox tea/water
Snack 2:	Handful (30 g) of Pumpkin seeds
Dinner:	Hippocrates Healing Soup
	1 cup detox tea/water
	1 large grapefruit

DAY 6

	1 cup of Lemon-Ginger water
Breakfast:	Green Honeydew Smoothie
	1 cup detox tea/water
Snack 1:	10 carrot sticks (70 g) + 3 tbsp. of Tahini spread
Lunch:	Green Honeydew Smoothie
	1 cup detox tea/water
Snack 2:	1 Grapefruit, large (330 g) +
	60 g of sunflower seeds, roasted
Dinner:	Hippocrates Healing Soup
	1 cup detox tea/water
	1 medium sized apple

DAY 7

	1 cup of Lemon-Ginger water
Breakfast:	Green Mango Kale Smoothie
	1 cup detox tea/water
Snack 1:	30 g or 1 oz. of pumpkin or mixed seeds
Lunch:	Green Mango Kale Smoothie
	1 cup detox tea/water
Snack 2:	10 carrot sticks + 2 tbsp. of Tahini spread
Dinner:	Congee Chinese Rice Porridge with Cucumber Dill Salad
	1 cup detox tea/water

WEEK 3
7 DAY TRANSITION "POST-CLEANSE PHASE"

In this phase, you slowly going to transition from cleanse and fast to more solid foods and then back to a healthy diet and lifestyle. Week 3 of the 7 Day Transition "Post-Cleanse Phase"- Meal Plans are included for Vegan diet (strictly vegan) and Flexitarian diet (includes meat, fish, etc.). Choose one or the other, whichever is right for you. In this phase, you drink 1 fresh homemade smoothie daily, eat 2 meals with 2 snacks in between. You can snack on celery, carrots, cauliflower, cucumbers, apples, avocado, grapefruit if you get hungry. Also, on day 1-4 you can use a handful of unsalted seeds like pumpkin seeds, sunflower seeds, chia seeds, flax seeds, walnuts or almonds (omit if you are allergic to nuts).

You should be mindful of adding foods after the cleanse that enhance the detoxification process and support liver and kidney function. Some of the best foods for liver support include garlic, cruciferous vegetables like broccoli and broccoli sprouts, avocados, turmeric, beets, bitter foods like dandelion, chicory and arugula, and most leafy greens and fresh herbs.

Foods that support kidney function include onions and garlic, cranberries, cherries, lemon and lemon water, bell peppers, grapefruit, and celery. Of course, the best thing you can do for your kidneys is drink plenty of fresh, filtered water. Adequate hydration is critical for healthy kidneys, not to mention the rest of your body!

As you're cleansing, your digestive system was going through a rapid healing process. 'Breaking' the cleanse or returning to regular eating pattern must be done gradually and mindfully. Because animal products are very difficult to digest, and are mostly acidic, avoiding animal products of all kinds for at least 1 week before and after is recommended. This will ensure you maintain and assimilate the benefits of the cleanse you have just finished. It will also help you avoid any digestive distress you may experience from transitioning too quickly. After a week or two you may begin to add in small amounts of pastured animal products, but they should never be the main focus of the meal. Your meals should consist primarily of vegetables, fruits, sprouted grains, legumes, nuts and seeds, and small portions of animal products now and then.

In a world bombarded with more chemicals and toxins than ever before, it's easy to feel helpless and overwhelmed. Yet, we have the power to heal with every meal we choose. By cleansing and detoxing a few times each year, you are helping to support your body in substantial ways. **Above all, practice gratitude with every meal, enjoy your food, and share it with the people you love!**

WEEK 3. 7 DAY TRANSITION "POST-CLEANSE PHASE" VEGAN SHOPPING LIST

FRUITS
Apple, large 2
Apple, small, 1
Banana, medium 1
Cantaloupe (260 g)
Green grapes (160 g)
Kiwi fruit, 1
Lemon, 2
Lime, 1
Orange, 1 (140 g)
Papaya, (75 g)

SPICES & HERBS
Basil
Bay leaf
Black pepper
Cayenne pepper
Cilantro, fresh, 6 tbsp.
Coriander, ground
Cumin, ground
Italian spice mix
 Oregano
Parsley Fresh 4 tbsp.
rosemary, fresh 2 tbsp.
dill, fresh, 1 tbsp.
garlic powder
Onion powder
Nutmeg
Cinnamon
Smoked paprika
Thyme
Turmeric

STAPLES
Apple cider vinegar
Coconut oil
Flax seeds oil
Kosher salt,
Liquid smoke
Olive oil
Rice vinegar
Sesame oil
Sherry vinegar

FROZEN FOODS
Blueberries (510 g)
Mixed berries (510 g)
Pineapple chunks
(210 g)
Mango, chunks (85g)
Strawberries (130 g)

DRIED FRUIT, NUTS & SEEDS
Almonds, toasted, 0.5 oz.
Cashews 2 tbsp.
Chia seeds (60 g) or 2 oz.
Coconut flaxes, ¼ cup
Cranberries (8 g) 1 tbsp.
medjool dates, pitted, 3
Pumpkin or mixed seeds
(30 g)
Flaxseed, ground 120 g
Sesame seeds 1.5 oz.
Sunflower seeds 2 tbsp.
Walnuts 60g or 2 oz.

CANNED/ PACKAGED ITEMS
Almond milk, unsweetened
3 cups
Black beans, canned 34 oz.
Black-Olive-Spread
Chia bread
Chickpeas, 1-14 oz. cans
Cocoa powder, 1 tbsp.,
unsweetened
Coconut milk 1 cup
Coconut milk powder 4
tbsp.
Coconut yogurt 2.2 cups
Coconut, raw, shredded 2
oz. (60 g)
Crispy tofu cubes 5 oz. + 3
oz. of extra-firm tofu
Curry paste, 2 tbsp.
Hummus 1 tbsp.
Pinto beans, 10 oz.
Power Shot Greens

GRAINS& PRODUCTS
Rice short Grain (200 g)
oatmeal (120 g)
Quinoa, (85 g)
Cornstarch (60 g)
Amaranth (24 g)

VEGETABLES
Arugula 60 g
Asparagus spears, 6
Beet, small 1
Bell Pepper, 2
Bok Choy, (420 g)
Carrots medium 10
Cauliflower, (270 g)
Celery medium, 6
Cucumber, medium 3
(300 g)
Garlic, 15 cloves
Ginger, 1 root
Green onion, 2
Lettuce leaves, large
2 + 2 cups
Eggplant, 2 small
~1.8 lb.
Onion Red, medium 2
Mushrooms, Shiitake
dried 7 (125 g)
Mushrooms, white(70 g)
Greens mixed (30 g)
Onion, medium, 5
Peas (60 g)
Radishes, 5
Red pepper, roasted 4
Scallions, 4
Shallots 2
Spinach (240 g)
Zucchini, 2 lb.
Lentils (90 g) or 3 oz.
Kale (40 g)
Tomatoes, medium 4

WEEK 3. 7 DAY TRANSITION "POST-CLEANSE PHASE" VEGAN WEEKLY MEAL PLAN

	DAY 1	DAY 2	DAY 3	DAY 4	DAY 5	DAY 6	DAY 7
I MEAL	1 cup Lemon-Ginger drink or Water or Detox tea	1 cup Lemon-Ginger drink or Water or Detox tea	1 cup Lemon-Ginger drink or Water or Detox tea	1 cup Lemon-Ginger drink or Water or Detox tea	1 cup Lemon-Ginger drink or Water or Detox tea	1 cup Lemon-Ginger drink or Water or Detox tea	1 cup Lemon-Ginger drink or Water or Detox tea
	1 serving of Green Probiotics Smoothie	1 serving of Green Bliss Smoothie	1 serving Green Cantaloupe Berry Smoothie	1 serving Green Banana Coconut Smoothie	1 serving Green Kiwi Berry Smoothie	1 serving Green Berry Cucumber Smoothie	1 serving Green Enzyme Smoothie
SNACK	1 oz. Pumpkin seeds or mixed seeds	½ cup Coconut Yogurt w/ 1 oz. of chia + ½ cup of berries	10 carrot sticks	1 cup of mixed berries	½ cup blueberries	Energy ball (half amount of prepared balls)	1 serving of Amaranth pudding with coconut
II MEAL	1 cup Detox Tea/Water	1 cup Detox Tea/Water	1 cup Detox Tea/Water	1 cup Detox Tea/Water	1 cup Detox Tea/Water	1 cup Detox Tea/Water	1 cup Detox Tea/Water
	Seaweed Congee "Chinese Rice Porridge" w/ Cucumber Dill Salad	1 serving Grilled Veggie Wrap	1 serving Thai Curry Zucchini Soup/ Raw Beet Salad with seeds	1 serving of Bean Soup and Green Salad	1 serving of Lentil Soup with Greens with 1 Baked Potato	1 serving of Rice Tortilla Wrap with veggies	1 serving of Hawaiian Tofu Poke Bowl
SNACK	½ cup blueberries	1 apple, large	10 celery sticks cut into strips +2 tbsp. of Tahini-Lemon spread	10-14 halves of walnuts (1 oz. or 30g)	1 apple, large	10 celery sticks cut into strips + 2 tbsp. Pico de Gallo	Cantaloupe wedge + 2 tbsp. of Tahini spread
III MEAL	1 cup Detox Tea/Water	1 cup Detox Tea/Water	1 cup Detox Tea/Water	1 cup Detox Tea/Water	1 cup Detox Tea/Water	1 cup Detox Tea/Water	1 cup Detox Tea/Water
	2 servings Cranberry Cilantro Quinoa Salad	1 serving of Thai Curry Zucchini Soup	1 serving of Bean Soup with Grilled Veggies	1 serving of Lentil Soup with Greens with Green Salad	1 serving Tomato, Cauliflower & Spinach Curry	1 serving of Vegan Chili with 1 Baked Potato	1 serving Vegan Chickpea Meatloaf with Mushroom Gravy and Steamed Broccoli
whole day kcal	whole day kcal	whole day kcal	whole day kcal	whole day kcal	whole day kcal	whole day kcal
1127	1121	1424	1292	1547	1223	1462

WEEKLY AVERAGE 1320 KCAL PER DAY

WEEK 3. 7 DAY TRANSITION "POST-CLEANSE PHASE" VEGAN WEEKLY MEAL PLAN

DAY 1

	1 cup of Lemon-Ginger /Water
Breakfast:	Green Probiotic Smoothie
	1 cup detox tea/water
Snack 1:	30 g or 1oz. pumpkin seeds or mixed seeds
Lunch:	Seaweed Congee "Chinese Rice Porridge" with Cucumber Dill Salad
	1 cup detox tea/water
Snack 2:	1 cup blueberries (75g)
Dinner:	Cranberry Cilantro Quinoa Salad
	1 cup detox tea/water

DAY 2

	1 cup of Lemon-Ginger /water
Breakfast:	Green Bliss Smoothie
	1 cup detox tea/water
Snack 1:	½ cup coconut yogurt with 1 oz. of chia + ½ cup of berries
Lunch:	Grilled Veggie Wrap
	1 cup detox tea/water
Snack 2:	1 apple, large
Dinner:	Thai Curry Zucchini Soup
	1 cup detox tea/water

DAY 3

	1 cup of Lemon-Ginger water
Breakfast:	Green Cantaloupe Berry Smoothie
	1 cup detox tea/water
Snack 1:	10 carrot sticks (70 g)
Lunch:	Thai Curried Zucchini Soup/Raw Beet Salad with seeds
	1 cup detox tea/water
Snack 2:	10 celery sticks cut into strips + 2 tbsp. of Tahini-Lemon spread
Dinner:	Bean Soup with Grilled Veggies
	1 cup detox tea/water

DAY 4

Breakfast:
1 cup of Lemon-Ginger /Water
Green Banana Coconut Smoothie
1 cup detox tea/water

Snack 1: 1 cup of mixed berries
Lunch: Bean Soup with Green Salad
1 cup detox tea/water

Snack 2: 10-14 halves of walnuts (1 oz. or 30 g)
Dinner: Lentil Soup with Green Salad
1 cup detox tea/water

DAY 5

Breakfast:
1 cup of Lemon-Ginger /water
Green Kiwi Berry Smoothie
1 cup detox tea/water

Snack 1: ½ cup Coconut Yogurt w/ Chia + ½ cup Blueberries
Lunch: Lentil Soup (1 serving) with 1 Baked Potato (160 g)
1 cup detox tea/water

Snack 2: Chia bread + 2 tbsp. of Black Olive Spread
Dinner: Tomato, Cauliflower & Spinach Curry

1 cup detox tea/water

DAY 6

Breakfast:
1 cup of Lemon-Ginger water
Green Cucumber Smoothie
1 cup detox tea/water

Snack 1: Energy ball (half amount of prepared balls)
Lunch: Rice Tortilla Wrap with Veggies
1 cup detox tea/water

Snack 2: 1 apple, large + 2 tbsp. of Tahini Lemon Spread
Dinner: Vegan Chili + 1 Baked Potato (160 g)

1 cup detox tea/water

DAY 7

Breakfast:
1 cup of Lemon-Ginger water
Green Enzyme Smoothie
1 cup detox tea/water

Snack 1: Amaranth pudding with coconut
Lunch: Hawaiian Poke Bowl
1 cup detox tea/water

Snack 2: Cantaloupe wedge (100 g) + 2 tbsp. of Tahini spread
Dinner: Vegan Chickpea Meatloaf with
Mushroom Gravy and Steamed Broccoli
1 cup detox tea/water

WEEK 3. 7 DAY TRANSITION "POST-CLEANSE PHASE" FLEXITARIAN SHOPPING LIST

FRUITS
Blueberries (360 g)
Apple, large 2
Apple, small 1
Cantaloupe wedge (180 g)
Grapes green (160 g) or 1 cup Banana, medium 1
Kiwi fruit, 1
Strawberries (130 g)
Papaya (75 g)
Orange, 1 (140 g)
Lime 2
Lemon 3

FROZEN FOODS
Mixed berries (290 g)
Pineapple chunks (210 g)
Mango chunks (85 g)
Sour cherries (60 g)
Salmon, wild, filet 7 oz.
Chicken thighs (300 g)
Turkey ground (90 g)

CANNED/ PACKAGED ITEMS
Almond milk 1.5 cup
Coconut yogurt 2 cups
Coconut milk 350 ml
Coconut flakes, shredded 120 g
Coconut Milk Powder 5 tbsp.
Tahini-Lemon spread 4 tbsp. Pico de Gallo 2 tbsp. (30 g) Power Shot Greens Superfood powder 7 tbsp.
Tofu Crispy cubes 5 oz., firm 3 oz.
Hummus 1 tbsp.
Thai Curry Paste 2 tbsp.
Vegetable broth 8 cups
black Beans, canned 30 oz.
Basil-pesto-hummus
Chicken broth 4 cups
Tomatoes Canned 17 oz.
Pinto beans, canned 9 oz.

DRIED FRUIT, NUTS & SEEDS
Dried cranberries 1
tPumpkin seeds (60 g)
Chia seeds (30 g)
Walnuts (50 g)
Flaxseed 6 tbsp.
Cranberries 1 tbsp.
Almonds 1 tbsp.
Sesame seeds (60 g)
Dates, 3

STAPLES
Vanilla powder
Olive oil
Salt
Apple cider Vinegar
Coconut oil
Cocoa powder
Sherry vinegar
Vegan ground meat (optional) ½ -1 cup reduced-sodium tamari
Sesame oil
Rice vinegar

SPICES & HERBS
Black pepper
Red pepper
Cumin
Dill
coriander
Thyme
Oregano
Italian spice mix,
Turmeric,
Cinnamon
1 bay leaf

GRAINS& PRODUCTS
Rice short grain (160 g)
Quinoa, (85 g)
Amaranth (24 g)

VEGETABLES
Arugula 30g
Bell pepper 3 (450 g)
Bell Pepper, roasted, 6
Cabbage, (70 g)
Carrot, medium, 13
Celery, medium, 10
Cucumber, (650 g)
Cilantro, fresh 5 tbsp.
Tomato, medium 5(580 g)
Lettuce 2 large leaves +1 cup
Eggplant, medium,1 (460 g)
Onion red, 2
Onion, yellow, medium 6
Garlic, 18 cloves
Mushrooms, shiitake dried 7 or 125 g
Bok Choy, (420 g)
Ginger, small 1
Green onion, 2
Leek, smaller, (45 g)
Lentils (90 g) 3 oz.
Kale (40 g)
Olives (60 g)
Parsley 1 tbsp.
Radishes, 5,
Peas (60 g)
Potatoes, medium 2 (430 g)
Scallions 6
Shallots, small, 2(40 g)
Spinach (90 g)
Zucchini, 1.7 lb.

WEEK 3: 7 DAY TRANSITION "POST-CLEANSE PHASE" FLEXITARIAN WEEKLY MEAL PLAN

	DAY 1	DAY 2	DAY 3	DAY 4	DAY 5	DAY 6	DAY 7
I MEAL	1 cup Lemon-Ginger drink or Water or Detox tea	1 cup Lemon-Ginger drink or Water or Detox tea	1 cup Lemon-Ginger drink or Water or Detox tea	1 cup Lemon-Ginger drink or Water or Detox tea	1 cup Lemon-Ginger drink or Water or Detox tea	1 cup Lemon-Ginger drink or Water or Detox tea	1 cup Lemon-Ginger drink or Water or Detox tea
	1 serving of Green Probiotics Smoothie	1 serving Green Bliss Smoothie	1 serving Green Cantaloupe Berry Smoothie	1 serving Green Banana Coconut Smoothie	1 serving Green Kiwi Berry Smoothie	1 serving Green Berry Cucumber Smoothie	1 serving Green Enzyme Smoothie
SNACK	1 oz. Pumpkin seeds or mixed seeds	½ cup Coconut Yogurt w/ 1 oz. of chia + ½ cup of berries	10 carrot sticks	1 cup of mixed berries	½ cup blueberries	Energy ball (half amount of prepared balls)	1 serving of Amaranth pudding with coconut
II MEAL	1 cup Detox Tea/Water	1 cup Detox Tea/Water	1 cup Detox Tea/Water	1 cup Detox Tea/Water	1 cup Detox Tea/Water	1 cup Detox Tea/Water	1 cup Detox Tea/Water
	Seaweed Congee Chinese Rice Porridge w/ Cucumber Dill Salad	1 serving of Grilled Veggie Wrap	1 serving of Thai Curry Zucchini Soup/ Asian Salad	1 serving Bean Soup with Green Salad	1 serving Grilled Wild Salmon, with Grilled Veggies	1 serving of Lemon Chicken Soup with Greek Salad	1 serving Hawaiian Tofu Poke Bowl
SNACK	½ cup blueberries	1 apple, large	10 celery sticks cut into strips +2 tbsp. of Tahini-Lemon spread	10-14 halves of walnuts (1 oz. or 30g)	1 apple, large	10 celery sticks cut into strips + 2 tbsp. Pico de Gallo	Cantaloupe wedge + 2 tbsp. of Tahini spread
III MEAL	1 cup Detox Tea/Water	1 cup Detox Tea/Water	1 cup Detox Tea/Water	1 cup Detox Tea/Water	1 cup Detox Tea/Water	1 cup Detox Tea/Water	1 cup Detox Tea/Water
	double serving of Cranberry Cilantro Quinoa Salad	1 serving Thai Curry Zucchini Soup	1 serving of Bean Soup with Grilled Veggies	1 serving of Lentil Soup with Greens with Green Salad	1 serving Lemon Chicken Soup	1 serving Vegan Chili	1 serving Stuffed Bell Peppers with Ground Turkey

whole day kcal	whole day kcal	whole day kcal	whole day kcal	whole day kcal	whole day kcal	whole day kcal
1127	1217	1460	1292	1548	1274	1486

WEEKLY AVERAGE 1453 KCAL PER DAY

WEEK 3: 7 DAY TRANSITION "POST-CLEANSE PHASE" FLEXITARIAN WEEKLY MEAL PLAN

DAY 1

	1 cup of Lemon-Ginger /Water
Breakfast:	Green Probiotics Smoothie
	1 cup detox tea/water
Snack 1:	30 g or 1 oz. of Pumpkin seeds or mixed seeds
Lunch:	Seaweed Congee Chinese Rice Porridge with Cucumber Dill Salad
	1 cup detox tea/water
Snack 2:	½ cup blueberries
Dinner:	Cranberry Cilantro Quinoa Salad
	1 cup detox tea/water

DAY 2

	1 cup of Lemon-Ginger /water
Breakfast:	Green Bliss Smoothie
	1 cup detox tea/water
Snack 1:	½ cup Coconut Yogurt w/ 1 oz. of chia + ½ cup of berries
Lunch:	Grilled Veggie Wrap
	1 cup detox tea/water
Snack 2:	1 apple, large
Dinner:	Thai Curry Zucchini Soup
	1 cup detox tea/water

DAY 3

	1 cup of Lemon-Ginger water
Breakfast:	Green Cantaloupe Berry Smoothie
	1 cup detox tea/water
Snack 1:	10 carrot sticks
Lunch:	Thai Curry Zucchini Soup with Asian Salad
	1 cup detox tea/water
Snack 2:	10 celery sticks cut into strips + 2 tbsp. of Tahini-Lemon spread
Dinner:	Bean Soup with Grilled Veggies
	1 cup detox tea/water

DAY 4

	1 cup of Lemon-Ginger /Water
Breakfast:	Green Banana Coconut Smoothie
	1 cup detox tea/water
Snack 1:	1 cup of mixed berries
Lunch:	Bean Soup with Green Salad
	1 cup detox tea/water
Snack 2:	(1 oz. or 30 g) 10-14 halves of walnuts
Dinner:	Lentil Soup with Green Salad
	1 cup detox tea/water

DAY 5

	1 cup of Lemon-Ginger /water
Breakfast:	Green Kiwi Berry Smoothie
	1 cup detox tea/water
Snack 1:	½ cup blueberries (80 g)
Lunch:	Grilled Wild Salmon with Grilled Veggies
	1 cup detox tea/water
Snack 2:	1 apple, large (160 g)
Dinner:	Lemon Chicken Soup
o	1 cup detox tea/water

DAY 6

	1 cup of Lemon-Ginger water
Breakfast:	Green Berry Cucumber Smoothie
	1 cup detox tea/water
Snack 1:	Energy ball (half amount of prepared balls)
Lunch:	Lemon Chicken Soup with Greek Salad
	1 cup detox tea/water
Snack 2:	10 celery sticks cut into strips (40g) +
	2 tbsp. Pico de Gallo (30 g)
Dinner:	Vegan Chili
	1 cup detox tea/water

DAY 7

	1 cup of Lemon-Ginger water
Breakfast:	Green Enzyme Smoothie
	1 cup detox tea/water
Snack 1:	Amaranth pudding with coconut
Lunch:	Hawaiian Tofu Poke Bowl
	1 cup detox tea/water
Snack 2:	Cantaloupe wedge (100 g) + 2 tbsp. of Tahini spread
Dinner:	Stuffed Bell Pepper with Ground Turkey
	1 cup detox tea/water

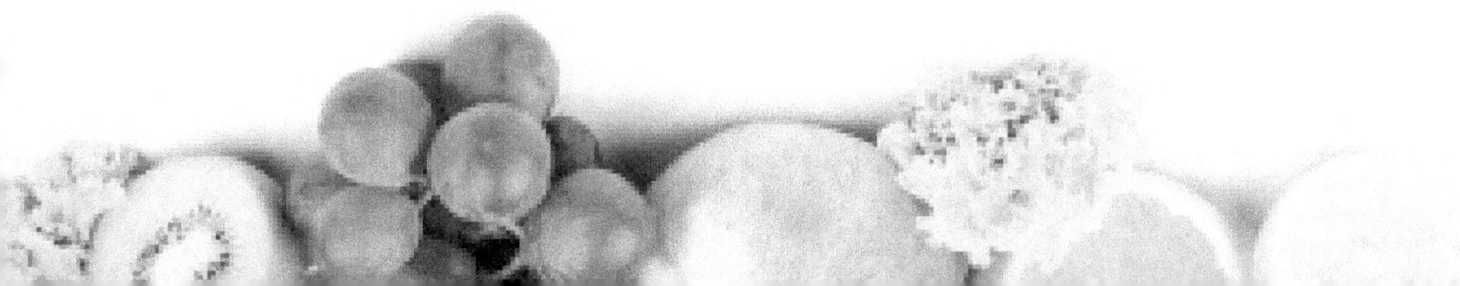

7 DAY GREEN SUPERFOOD SMOOTHIE CLEANSE Q AND A

CAN I LOSE WEIGHT DRINKING GREEN SUPERFOOD SMOOTHIES?

Yes. Drink your green smoothie as a replacement meal for one or two meals each day. You can follow this regimen for however long you need to reach your weight loss goal. Avoid adding too many fruits to each smoothie and use more fresh veggies which are full of fiber.

HOW CAN I GET MORE PROTEIN, IRON, AND CALCIUM IN MY SMOOTHIES?

If you are deficient in these nutrients, Green Smoothies are a great option because they chock full of nutrients, protein, trace minerals and iron.

WHY DO I SOMETIMES GET GAS AND BLOATING AFTER MY GREEN SUPERFOOD SMOOTHIE?

If you've been eating a steady diet high in refined or processed foods, drinking a blended Green Smoothie full of raw fruits and greens can be a bit of a shock to your digestive system. Your stomach may be low in digestive acids, or you may have an imbalance of gut bacteria. The can result is excess gas and bloating as your stomach tries to correct itself and find a healthy balance.

DO I HAVE TO USE GREENS IN MY GREEN SUPERFOOD SMOOTHIE?

You should incorporate greens into each smoothie because the whole point of having a Green Smoothie is to get more leafy greens into your diet. The benefit of drinking your greens is that it's easy to do every day, takes less than 5 minutes to prepare, and tastes great!

WHAT IF I GET A STOMACH CRAMPS WHEN I DRINK MY GREEN SUPERFOOD SMOOTHIE?

You may be drinking your Green Smoothie too fast or too cold, or your smoothie is too sweet. You should always move it around in your mouth before swallowing. This gives you at least 2 benefits. The first is that it gets to be mixed with your saliva which aids in digestion. The second is that it will warm your smoothie so it is more readily accepted by your stomach. Also, if it is too sweet, try adding a higher percentage of vegetables and less sweet fruits.

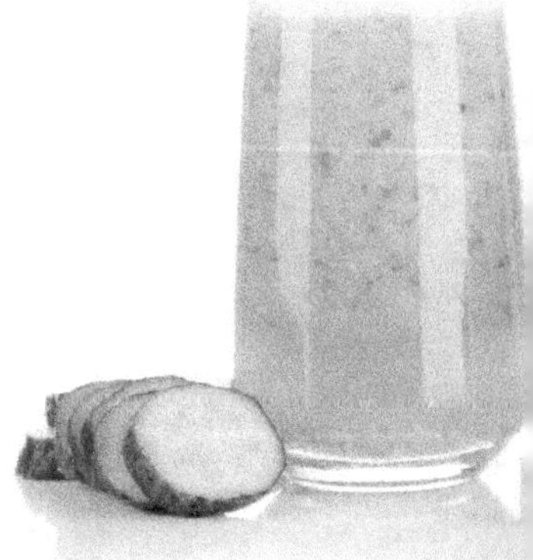

WHAT IS THE DIFFERENCE BETWEEN A GREEN SMOOTHIE AND A GREEN JUICE?

Both are great for your health! Rather, consider which one is more practical for your lifestyle. In terms of the health benefits, both green smoothies and green juices offer a vast array of minerals, vitamins, and chlorophyll. The biggest difference between the two is that green smoothies still have all fiber intact, whereas juice has no fiber

IS IT POSSIBLE TO DRINK TOO MANY GREEN SUPERFOOD SMOOTHIES?

Highly unlikely. Green Smoothies have a lot of natural fiber in them. Fiber fills you up and stops you from overeating. Also, your body will be getting a vast array of nutrients and will be nutritionally satisfied, and will not want more food.

DO GREEN SUPERFOOD SMOOTHIES WORK AGAINST CELLULITE?

The cause of cellulite is usually weak collagen, excess fat accumulation, and a buildup of toxins. As you age, collagen production declines and weakening of the skin occurs. Dark leafy green vegetables and a variety of fruits contain powerful antioxidants that naturally help your skin produce more collagen to help repair and rejuvenate your skin, and you'll quickly start seeing positive results.

DON'T GREEN SUPERFOOD SMOOTHIES TASTE LIKE GRASS?

No. The recipes in this book combine veggies and fruits to help balance and sweeten the flavor, and most people find that they taste delicious. The recipes are optimized for nutrition and taste. You can also experiment with creating your own smoothie masterpieces.

DO I NEED AN EXPENSIVE BLENDER TO MAKE GREEN SUPERFOOD SMOOTHIES?

The simple answer to this question is no, you can get started with any blender, however, with a high quality blender, you will get a smooth creamy result every time. But they cost a lot of money and you should remember that the most important thing is to get started, not having the perfect blender. You can always upgrade as you go.

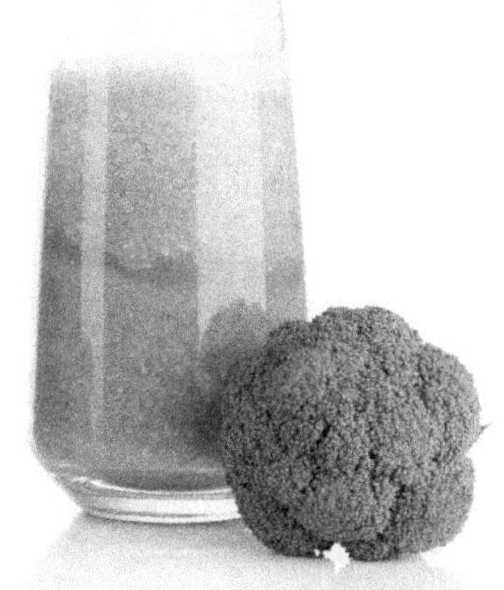

CAN I ADD SWEETENERS?
If you find that a recipe isn't sweet enough for your taste, simply add some more banana or other ripe fruits that offer a natural sweetness.

CAN I USE FROZEN FRUIT INSTEAD OF FRESH?
Yes, frozen fruits are fine to use. If you have some over-ripe fruit on hand, just freeze it in a plastic bag and use it when you need it instead of letting it go to waste. You can also buy bags of frozen fruit at the supermarket.

CAN I REPLACE A MEAL WITH A GREEN SUPERFOOD SMOOTHIE?
Yes, absolutely! This is an ideal way to have a nutritious meal at any time of the day. I like to have my smoothie in the morning as a breakfast meal. This is a great way to cut down on sugary cereals, bread and dairy products. A serving of about two cups (16 oz.) is a good portion size.

WHAT ARE SOME GOOD NON-DAIRY OPTIONS FOR MILK?
Nut and seed milks are great and can be made from almost any nut or seed. Almond milk is most common and you can also buy this ready-made. Soya milk and rice milk can also be used but almond milk has more nutrition. Coconut water is another great liquid.

WHY DO I NEED TO USE POWER SHOT GREEN SUPERFOODS IN MY GREEN SMOOTHIES?
Power Shot Green Superfoods blend is an integral part of cleansing and detox because it contains a vast array of 14 green superfoods, in specific proportions that will support your body through the cleanse. It is also convenient, tasty and easy to use. Can you imagine having to search for, and buy 14 diferent green superfoods to add to your smoothies? This formula has already been used for many years by thousands of people. See the testimonials on Amazon or at the end of this book.

HOW CAN I USE MY POWER SHOT GREENS SUPRERFOODS BLEND?
You can mix in water, juice, add to smoothies, non-dairy milk, chocolate drink, yogurt. It instantly dissolves and is easily absorbed in your body.

Detox Aids

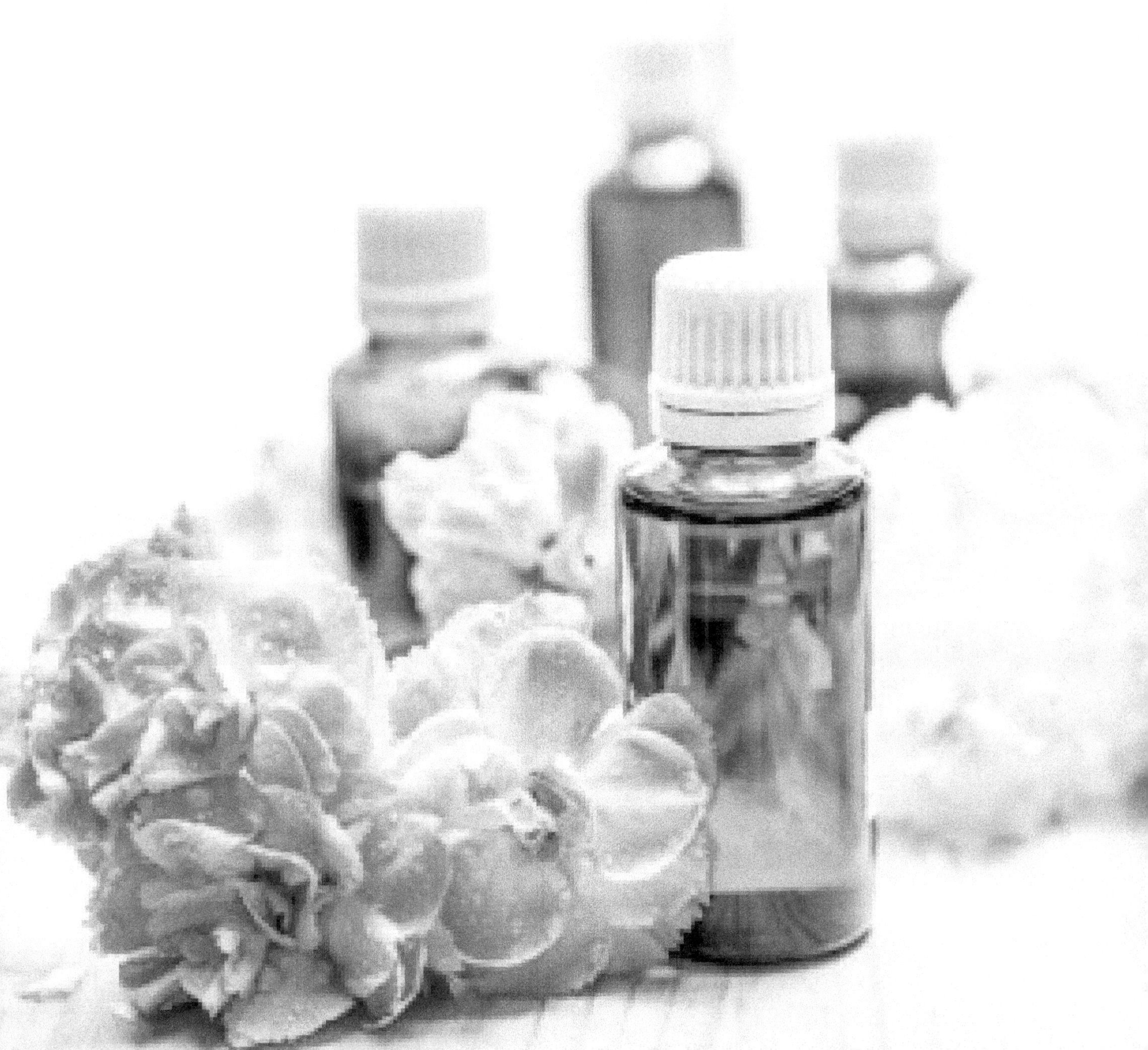

HELPFUL DETOX AIDS DURING FAST & CLEANSE

12 DETOXIFICATION STRATEGIES

When it comes to your cleanse and detox, having a wide variety of tools and knowledge is a huge plus. It can mean the difference between average results and great results. Thinking and doing things outside the normal scope of what you're currently implementing can take you to the next level.

Detox aids are designed to assist your body's natural cleansing and healing actions; they can speed up healing, recovery and help you get the most from your detox program! Below, we will discuss 12 different methods that will assist your detoxification efforts, and show you exactly how to use them for maximum benefit.

Some of these aids below require a qualified certified professional, health clinic, or spa.

1. COLON CLEANSING

A healthy colon is a vital part in the toxin-elimination process. Your bowels need to be clean and moving normally.
Here are a couple of treatments you may want to consider:

a) Enemas
Enemas have been part of medicine for thousands of years. The first reference of the use of enemas for health was by the Egyptians in 1550 BC. Greek physicians from the first century addressed health issues by prescribing healthy food, herbal drink, and enemas.

Enemas involve injecting liquid into the rectum, either for the purpose of introducing medication or for clearing out the contents of the bowels. There are different types if enema; cleansing, retention and herbal. The aim is to empty the bowels. Make sure you drink: 1 or 2 glasses of water before having an enema because sometimes Colon Cleansing can cause dehydration.

How do I do it?
Enema(s) procedure includes placing a rectal lubricated insertion nozzle into the rectum. Pour the solution into the enema bag and elevate the bag. Lie on your left side. The fluid will flow down gradually by gravity. Keep the enema bag no more than 2 feet above the level of your bottom. Absorbing the enema solution should take approximately 10 minutes. If you get cramps, slow down the flow by lowering the enema bag or squeeze the clamp. When the bag is empty, remove the tube and expel liquid in the toilet.

b) Coffee Enemas:
A coffee enema is a type of colon cleanse that involves injecting a brewed coffee liquid into your rectum, for the purpose of removing toxins. Two compounds in coffee, kahweol and cafestol palmitate are absorbed through the gut wall where they travels to your liver and stimulate the activity (up to 700%) of an enzyme called glutathione S-transferase (GST), a powerful detoxifying antioxidant which opens up the bile duct in your liver. This helps to release more bile from your liver to break down food components and moves them out of your body via the colon. By stimulating bile flow and the production of glutathione, this dramatically speeds up your detoxification process. Since the entire blood supply circulates through your liver every three minutes, it is important to retain the coffee for 12 to 15 minutes. In this case your blood circulates through your liver four to five times, removing toxins and purifying it much like "dialysis".
Use for: Headaches, sluggishness, tiredness, pain.

How do I do it?
When doing a coffee enema, it is imperative to use an appropriate coffee. You want to use a light roasted coffee that is free of mold and high in palmitic acid. Start by bringing 2 cups of filtered water to a boil. Add 1/2 tablespoon of coffee and turn down to simmer for 12 minutes. After 12 minutes, remove the liquid from the heat and let cool to body temperature. Once it has cooled, add the liquid to your enema bag. Lie on your left side and insert the enema tube a few inches inside the rectum. Use lubrication if needed. Once the tube is inserted, open the valve on the enema tube and rest calmly while the coffee fills the lower intestine. After all the coffee is inside, turn over and lay on the right side. Hold the coffee from 15-20 minutes, then void the liquid.

*Note, it may be difficult to hold two cups in the beginning. Start with ½ cup, and work your way up to two cups. Some people are extremely sensitive to caffeine, start with ½ tablespoon of coffee, and work your way up to 3 tablespoons if you tolerate it. Do this every day while cleansing, for up to one week. After that, a once-per-month maintenance enema is a good idea.

c) Colon Hydrotherapy:
Colon hydrotherapy, or 'colonic' is a method of inserting water into the bowels to flush out the colon. This can be helpful during your fast or cleanse to speed up the elimination of toxins, and to prevent them from being reabsorbed through the portal vein. A colonic is especially important in the case of constipation or slow transit times.

During the course of the colonic procedure a large volume of fluid up to [15 gallons may be introduced into the rectum (not all at once) unlike enemas, for which a small amount of fluid is used, While the water is entering your body through another tube fluids and waste are expelled. The procedure may be repeated several times until the colon is clean.

How do I do it?
Colon hydrotherapy is best done by a professional. Aim for once per week during your cleanse. Ask your therapist for recommendations for your specific situation.

2. COLON CLEANSING CASTOR OIL PACK
Castor oil is a thick, viscous oil obtained from the castor seed. The oil is known to boost the immune system, stimulate lymphatic drainage, and support liver detoxification. The beauty of the castor oil pack is that you put it directly onto the area you want to stimulate. So during your cleanse or fast, use a castor oil pack right over your liver to stimulate detoxification.

How do I do it?
To make the pack, source a good quality organic castor oil. Pour a small amount (about ¼ of a cup) onto a flannel cloth. Lay the cloth directly over your liver, and place a warm water bottle on top of the cloth. Rest calmly for about 30 minutes. This is best done right before bed. It is recommended to wear an old shirt that you don't mind getting dirty, the castor oil will stain.

3. HEALING AND DETOX WITH SAUNAS AND STEAM
The skin is the largest detoxifying organ in your body. Sweat analyses have shown heavy metals, hundreds of chemicals, pesticides, herbicides and other toxins excreted directly through the skin. Sweating is a very effective and very important detoxification process we should achieve at least several times per week. However, when we're participating in a cleanse, vigorous and strenuous exercise is not recommended. Instead, take advantage of sweat inducing saunas and steams to enhance your body's detoxification.

How do I do it?

a) Infrared Sauna:
Infrared saunas use either near or far infrared light spectrums to penetrate the skin and increase heating of your body. The light penetration effectively

causes your body to sweat. Reported benefits include stress relief, improved circulation, pain management, cardiovascular support, and of course, toxin elimination. You can purchase one for your home, or seek out a gym or treatment center. Use an infrared sauna at least 3 times per week for 15-20 minutes.

b) Steam Baths:

Used for millennia, steam baths have been an important part of many cultures' health practices across the globe. A steam bath is conducted in a dedicated room where the temperature is heated to about 115 degrees, and the humidity is at 100%. The combination of the heat and moisture helps to open up the pores, induce sweating, and helps to cleanse your body of those liberated toxins. Adding herbs to the steam like Eucalyptus is especially beneficial for respiratory conditions. Many gyms and health spas have steam rooms you can access.

4. DRY BRUSHING

Dry brushing your skin everyday helps to stimulate the lymphatic system to move waste through your body. It also enhances circulation, exfoliates the skin, and may reduce cellulite!

How do I do it?

First get yourself a natural bristle brush or loofah with firm texture. Begin on the bottoms of the feet, and gently brush in light strokes toward the heart. Work your way up your body, being extra gentle with the neck and chest. Avoid the face. This is best done before a bath or shower. Do at least 3 times per week, or everyday if possible.

5. TONGUE SCRAPING

It takes less than a minute and has significant health benefits. Scraping the tongue first thing in the morning removes the buildup of bacteria, yeast, chemicals, and plaque that has accumulated over night. This improves oral health and provides a manual cleansing of toxins that would have been swallowed otherwise.

How do I do it?

Purchase a good quality tongue scraper. Most health foods stores will sell them. Stainless steel scrapers are good options as they are non-toxic and very durable. Scrape the tongue from back to front about 10 times. Rinse off the scraper as much as needed. If you gag during the process, start a little higher up on the tongue. Do this every morning before brushing your teeth or consuming any foods or liquids.

6. BODY SCRUBS

A good body scrub consists of an exfoliating medium like salt or sugar, and a quality oil like jojoba, almond, grapeseed, or olive oil. Best done in the shower, a body scrub will help to exfoliate the skin, improve circulation and stimulate lymph movement. The oil leaves the skin incredibly soft and supple!

How do I do it?

There are many body scrubs on the market you can purchase. Make sure they use organic ingredients as much as possible. It is also very economical to make your own, and you can add essential oils to customize to your needs. A basic recipe consists of one part carrier oil to two parts salt and sugar. Add in a few drops of essential oil as desired. Once you have your scrub made, place it in the shower. In the middle of a hot shower, turn off the water and apply the scrub to legs, arms, and abdomen. Scrub gently in circular motions with light pressure. Turn water back on to rinse lightly, and towel off gently, so as not to remove all the oil.

7. CLAY WRAP AND PACKS

There are many different types of clays that can be applied topically. A clay 'wrap' or 'pack' is a certain type of clay that is placed directly on your skin. A wrap consists of applying the clay to the entire body and then wrapping your body in some kind of insulating shell like palm leaves, a thick sheet, or insulated blanket. A pack consists of applying the clay to one particular part of your body, the abdomen or liver, and then a warm cloth is placed over the specific location.

The benefits of wrapping or covering the clay are in the insulating effects. When your body is heated up, your pores are opened and thus the clay will have more drawing power. Clays have a strong adsorbing effect of toxins and heavy metals. When your pores are open, the clay will draw out more of the toxins directly through your skin. This makes the treatment a helpful addition for anyone having a 'cleansing or detoxing reaction'. Other benefits include pain management, swelling reduction, improvement in skin conditions, headache and nausea relief, and inflammation modulation.

How do I do it?

Start with sourcing a good quality clay. Popular choices include Bentonite, Montmorillonite, Pascalite, Dead Sea Clay, Red, or Green clay.
When performing this treatment, you have three options:

• Clay Wrap

First, dry brush your skin for a gentle exfoliation. Next make a paste from the dried clay powder and add a little bit of purified water. Add small amounts of water until you get a thick, yet pliable paste. Before applying to your body, you'll want to sit in the bathtub or an area where the floor and surrounding surfaces can get dirty. Apply the paste to all parts of your body- you may need a helper. Once all the paste is applied, wrap your body in a blanket, sheet, plastic wrap or other covering. Lay back and relax until all the clay feels dry. Remove the wrap and shower off all the clay. There are many spas and treatment centers that offer customized clay wraps. If you're not a DIY'er, this will be a good option for you.

• Clay Pack
As with the wrap, gently dry brush the specific body part you're going to apply the clay to. Most people use a clay pack on the abdomen and/or liver to help draw out toxins from those areas. It can also be used on areas that are injured or swollen, but take care not to apply to broken or irritated skin. After dry brushing, mix your clay with a small amount of water until you have a thick paste. You can either brush a cloth (a flannel or woolen cloth works well) with the clay, or apply the clay directly to your skin. Cover the area with a cloth, and put a hot water bottle on top. Relax until the clay is dry, and wash off.

• Clay Bath
With this method, you simply add a few cups of the clay to a warm bath and soak for 20-30 minutes. Be sure to use filtered water and rinse off completely when through.

All of these options can be done daily when completing a cleansing or detoxifying protocol. The elimination of the toxins directly through the skin will greatly enhance the cleansing process and help with any 'healing reactions' you may have.

8. MASSAGE
Who doesn't love a good massage? Not only does it feel amazing, but the health benefits are seemingly endless. Massage is one of the best stress relievers available. It also helps to move stagnant lymph, increase circulation, energize your body, relieve tension and knots in your muscles, improve sleep, reduce anxiety, modulate pain and inflammation, improve injuries, and lot more!

9. SALT CAVES OR ROOMS
Natural salt caves can be found across the globe. If you find yourself in Belarus or Slovakia for example, you can book a session in their specialized salt caves. You simply sit in the room for about 30 minutes and relax while you naturally inhale the salt into your lungs. 'Man-made' salt rooms are becoming more popular as well. These are usually made from Himalayan salt bricks and may have salt floors and salt lamps as well. Just like in the caves, you simply lay back and relax while inhaling the salted air.

10. SEA SALT BATHING OR OCEAN BATHING

Bathing in ocean waters has been a long standing 'prescription' by healers throughout the world. Reported benefits include detoxification, pain management, swelling reduction, and intense relaxation. The easiest way to take advantage of this treatment is to swim in the ocean. If you're not near ocean waters, you can simply add a cup or two of sea salt to a warm bath. Adding in magnesium or Epsom salts will provide additional benefit. Soak for at least 20 minutes. **This is best done right before bed.**

11. BODY WRAPS FOR CELLULITE AND WEIGHT LOSS

Body wraps involve applying essential oils, clays, seaweeds, herbs, minerals, or other plant material to your body, and then wrapping your body with plastic wrap, a sheet, or a blanket. Applying heat can be beneficial for opening the pores and increasing absorption of the medium applied.

How do I do it?

Gently exfoliate your skin via the dry brushing technique explained above. Next apply the chosen product to your entire body and wrap in the plastic wrap, sheet or blanket. Rest comfortably for 30 minutes to an hour, and remove the wrap. Rinse off well with warm water. Many professional spas offer this service.

12. HEALING AND DETOXIFYING WITH EXERCISE

Exercise is the ultimate lymphatic system cleanser. Your lymph system is responsible for moving fluids and waste throughout your entire body. Unlike the heart however, it does not have a pump. In order for lymph to move, you must move your body. Muscle contractions and joint movement is how lymph is stimulated to move.

Exercise is free, always available, and something you can do every day. Make sure you add some form of exercise to your protocol on a daily basis - just keep it light and gentle so as not to add too much stress on your body.

Some suggestions:

Walking, swimming, rebounding, bicycling, stretching, rowing. It doesn't matter what you do as long as you get up and move at least 20 minutes daily.

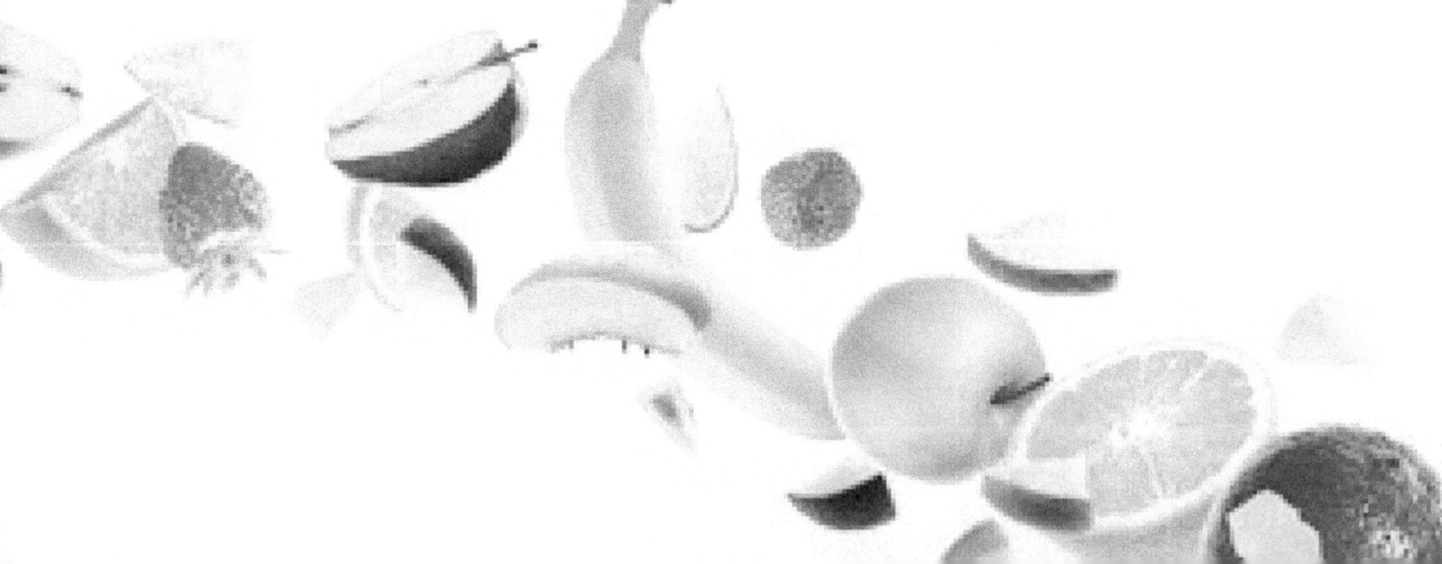

HEALING & DETOX WITH HERBAL REMEDIES AND ESSENTIAL OILS

Don't underestimate the power of simple 'every day' kitchen herbs that you may already have in the cupboard or yard. If you follow a whole foods diet, it's likely you have some of these powerhouses laying around. During your fast or cleanse is a great time to utilize their healing powers. There are many beneficial home herbal remedies.

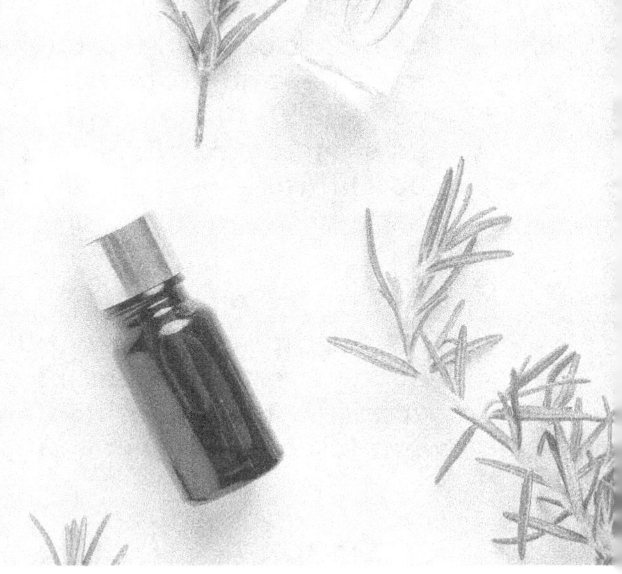

DANDELION
Commonly considered a pesky weed, dandelion is an amazing herb for supporting liver and detoxification. Kynurenic acid in abundant in dandelion which helps to stimulate bile production. The entire herb is rich in antioxidants and has a mild diuretic effect. Both are important for proper detoxification and elimination. Simply pick the weed, roots and all, and steep about ½ cup in boiling water. Drink several cups per day.

CILANTRO
This household herb is known for its excellent abilities to liberate heavy metals, especially mercury. You can put cut up cilantro into a tea, or take as a tincture. Be sure to drink extra water when using cilantro so that the liberated metals can be escorted out of your body.

GINGER
Ginger tea, tincture, capsules, or powder are all ways to consume this popular rhizome. Ginger is great for aiding detoxification due to its heating properties. Ginger stimulates digestion and circulation while warming your body and can even induce sweating. These actions will help to clear excess waste and buildup from your body. Whichever method of ingestion you choose, try to get about 3 servings of ginger per day.

LEMON

Drinking water with lemon first thing in the morning is a great way to stimulate digestion, encourage bile production and enhance liver function. Lemon is a rich source of citric acid, which has been shown to protect your liver and prevent oxidative damage. Add the juice of one fresh lemon to an eight-ounce glass of water. Drink first thing every morning.

MILK THISTLE

The most popular herb available for liver support, milk thistle reigns supreme for its hepatic protection. Milk thistle is rich in silymarin, and helps rebuild liver cells. It also helps to regenerate a damaged liver that is suffering from heavy metal toxicity, excessive alcohol consumption, or chemical exposure. You can take milk thistle in capsules, tea, or tinctures. It's best to take milk thistle between meals, three times per day.

ESSENTIAL OILS

The popularity of essential oils has increased substantially over the last decade. Certain essential oils have an affinity for liver and detoxification support. When choosing essential oils, make sure you trust the brand. If you want to consume them, only use essential oils labeled as food grade.

Good choices include:

- **LEMON :** As seen above, lemon helps to stimulate digestion and protect your liver. Add a few drops to your water bottle and drink throughout the day.
- **GRAPEFRUIT :** A lovely oil that smells great, grapefruit is uplifting and energizing. During a cleanse, it can be helpful to use grapefruit topically to move lymph and blood. Add about 5-10 drops in ½ cup carrier oil and use as massage oil during a full body massage.
- **LEMONGRASS :** This light and pleasant smelling oil is great for fluid drainage while doing a cleanse. Generally this oil can be applied directly to your skin, or added to a carrier oil. Use liberally.
- **GINGER :** Like the ginger root itself, ginger oil will aid circulation and support your body's detoxification efforts. Essential oil of ginger can be quite strong. Start with only a few drops added to a water bottle and drink throughout the day. Ginger can also be applied topically diluted in a carrier oil. Add a few drops to ½ cup carrier oil and apply as needed to your abdomen or liver.

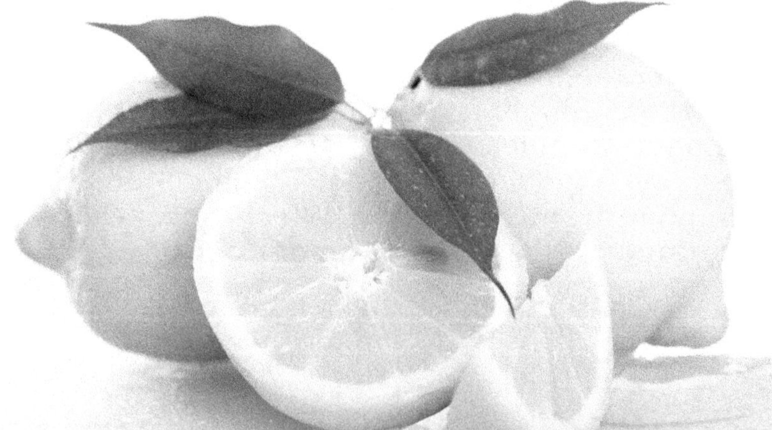

HEALING & DETOXING WITH SUPPLEMENTS

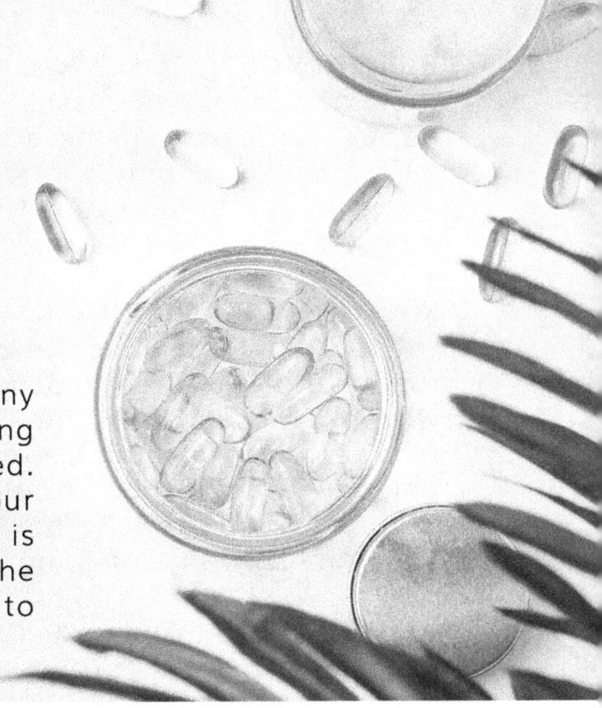

In an ideal world, you wouldn't need to take any supplements because you would get everything you need from the food and drinks you consumed. Unfortunately, in the modern world, we find our soil depleted, water contaminated, and the air is full of chemicals and toxins we breathe around the clock. Because of this, you need extra support to keep your body healthy.

Thankfully, we can take advantage of good quality supplements to balance out any deficiencies and help our body get rid of the chemical onslaught. During a cleanse, we need to support methylation, which is a process that converts toxic substances to water-soluble components so they can be easily excreted. We also need to support the organs of detoxification, namely, your liver, kidneys and gallbladder.

SUPPLEMENTS TO SUPPORT THE DETOXIFICATION PROCESS

GLUTATHIONE : The body's main detoxification and antioxidant. Glutathione is imperative for proper methylation and detoxification. Not all glutathione supplements are created equal. Liposomal glutathione seems to be the best absorbed. *Take 200-300mg on an empty stomach in the morning, and in the evening.*

SELENIUM : Selenium is a very important mineral that helps to bind and neutralize mercury. Most of us have traces of mercury in our bodies, if not more, due to the exposure in the air and water. *Take 100 mcg with each meal, or three times per day.*

MILK THISTLE : Rich in silymarin, milk thistle helps your liver produce glutathione, thus enhancing detoxification and methylation. *Take 200 mg between meals twice daily.*

B VITAMINS : The B vitamin family directly contributes to methylation (detoxification) processes throughout your body. Methylation will not happen efficiently if there is a deficiency in the B vitamins, specifically B6, B12, riboflavin, niacin and folate. A good quality food-based b-complex will support adequate methylation. Make sure the B12 and folate are in a methylated form. *Take once per day.*

MAGNESIUM AND ZINC : Mineral balancing is key for effective methylation to occur. Of particular importance are magnesium and zinc. Responsible for several hundred biochemical processes in your body, supplementing with magnesium and zinc is a good idea. Supplement with a good quality magnesium like magnesium gluconate or malate. Take 200 mg two times per day. Zinc can be supplemented in doses around 25 mg once per day. Copper is important to balance out zinc, so you may want to choose a zinc supplement with 1 or 2 mg of copper added.

AMINO ACIDS : Amino acids are what make up glutathione, and encourage proper methylation processes. Your liver will have to work hard to detoxify adequately without an abundant supply of amino acids. Supplementing with high quality essential amino acids during a fast or cleanse is a smart idea.

SUPPLEMENTS TO SUPPORT THE GI MICROBIOME

MODIFIED CITRUS PECTIN : MCP is a form of soluble fiber made from the rind, seeds and pith of citrus fruits. It has an affinity for binding to both cholesterol and heavy metals. The fiber itself helps to feed good bacteria in the gut, making this supplement a powerhouse for your cleansing protocol. Take ½ teaspoon in 8 ounces of water. Work your way up to 3 teaspoons if well tolerated and bowels are moving freely. *Take every day during your cleanse.*

DIGESTIVE ENZYMES : Digestive enzymes are important for anyone that has GI distress after eating. If you ever experience gas, bloating, indigestion or fatigue after meals, you may need enzymes to help support digestion. *Take 1-2 capsules with each meal.* These can also be taken in between meals to help assist inflammation and the cleanup of cellular debris.

PROBIOTICS : You've certainly heard of probiotics and the importance of probiotics in supporting your GI health. Both probiotic rich foods and supplements can be helpful if you suffer from any GI issues. When choosing a supplement, make sure it has at least 6-7 different strains, the more the better. *Take 1 to 2 capsules with the biggest meal of the day.*

ALOE VERA : Aloe Vera has a number of health benefits. Its mucilaginous properties make it an excellent supplement for soothing an inflamed digestive tract and feeding the good bacteria at the same time. Full of minerals and amino acids, aloe juice or gel is a great addition to any health routine. Take 1 tbsp. once per day. May be taken straight, or diluted in water or juice.

APPLE CIDER VINEGAR : Apple cider vinegar is a great digestive stimulant. When taken before a meal, it stimulates stomach acid production. This helps to digest food and kill any harmful microbes that may be hiding in your meal. ACV also helps to balance blood sugar, and is a good source of probiotics due to the fermentation process. Take 1 tablespoon diluted in 4-8 ounces of water before each meal, or first thing in the morning on an empty stomach.

SUPPLEMENTS TO SUPPORT COLON CLEANSE

ACTIVATED CHARCOAL : Charcoal has impressive adsorbing properties of toxins, heavy metals, and unwanted microbes. Taking charcoal during a cleanse will help to bind to these substances so they are not recirculated in your body. Take 2-3 capsules on an empty stomach with 16 ounces of water once per day. If constipation or slow bowels result, drop back to a lower dose.

BENTONITE CLAY : Also known for its absorbent properties, bentonite clay will help bind heavy metals and the liberated toxins from your fat stores. Follow the direction on the package.

LIQUID CHLOROPHYLL : Sometimes referred to as 'green gold,' liquid chlorophyll has amazing health benefits. Of particular interest is its ability to bind to carcinogens and prevent them from being absorbed in the digestive tract. For this reason it's a great addition to any fast or cleansing program. Take 100 mg, 3 times per day with meals.

NIACIN : A member of the B-vitamin family, Niacin has long been used to support cardiovascular health, balance blood sugar, and support detoxification. When taken in a supplement form, Niacin causes dilation of the blood vessels, enhancing blood flow and increasing detoxification. Take 500 mg once per day with a full meal.
Note, Niacin causes a 'flushing' reaction in many people. It is harmless, but can be alarming if you don't know what it is.

SUPPLEMENTS TO SUPPORT COLON HEALTH

PSYLLIUM HUSKS : We all know how important fiber is for our health, but few of us get enough in our diets. Supplementing with psyllium husks is an easy way to ensure you're getting what you need. Psyllium husks come from the Plantago ovate plant. It is rich in soluble fiber and expands when it's mixed in water. When ingested, it absorbs toxins and gently brushes the colon of debris and waste. Mix 1 tablespoon in 8 ounces of water and drink immediately. *Take 1 to 2 times per day, backing off the dose slightly if gas or constipation occurs.*

CASCARA SAGRADA : Cascara Sagrada is the dried bark of Rhamnus pushiana tree. It contains compounds called anthraquinones which have strong laxative effects. During a cleanse, it is imperative to keep bowels moving at least 1-3 times per day. If you need to speed up transit time or bowel movements, take Cascara Sagrada in tea, powder, or capsules. Follow the instructions on the bottle as potency varies.

MAGNESIUM : Different forms of magnesium have different properties. Magnesium oxide for example, is great at causing loose bowels. If you need to encourage a bowel movement, taking 400 mg of magnesium oxide can do the trick. Take before bed to encourage a morning bowel movement. Increase or decrease the dose until you reach your desired benefits.

SUPPLEMENTS TO SUPPORT LIVER AND GALL BLADDER HEALTH

APPLE JUICE : Freshly squeezed apple juice is full of malic acid. Malic acid helps to thin the bile. Keeping bile flow moving is very important during a cleanse. If bile is thick or sluggish, your liver can get backed up, and obviously you don't want that. Drink the juice of one juiced apple every day on an empty stomach for one week prior to beginning your cleanse. You can continue throughout the cleanse if you'd like, but be aware of the sugar content.

BEET TABLETS, POWDER, OR JUICE : Beets are another source of malic acid. If you don't like beets, you can buy beet tablets, powders or juices. You can add the powders and juices to smoothies or soups to dilute the taste. Capsules would provide the most convenience. Follow manufacturer recommendations.

MALIC ACID : If you don't like the idea of apple juice or beets, or you're concerned about the sugar content, you can take malic acid in supplement form. Take 500 mg once per day with a meal.

OX BILE : Just like it sounds, ox bile is a supplement made from the bile of oxen. If you have had your gall bladder removed, or you suffer from gallstones, supplementing with ox bile will replace the lack of bile you may experience. This will help with fat emulsification and absorption, and reduce GI distress like gas and bloating. Not needed if you are vegan or vegetarian

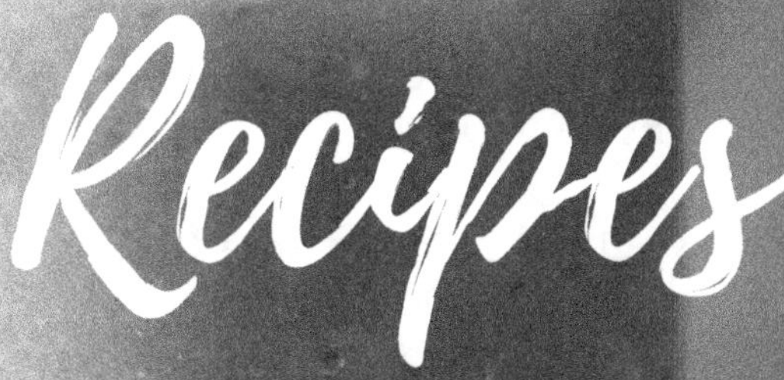
Recipes

Breakfast Recipes

Green Enzyme Smoothie

Servings: 1
Serving Size: 480 g or 16.9 oz.
Preparation time: 5 minutes

INGREDIENTS:
½ cup papaya, frozen chunks (75 g)
½ cup pineapple, frozen chunks (85 g)
1 navel orange, peeled (140 g)
1 tbsp. Power Shot Greens Superfood powder
1 tbsp. Coconut Milk Powder
½ cup water or unsweetened almond milk

DIRECTIONS: Blend and enjoy!

NUTRITIONAL INFORMATION

Energy (calories): 260kcal
Protein: 7.13 g
Fats: 5.97 g
Carbohydrates: 51.24 g
Fiber: 7.32 g

Green Banana Coconut Smoothie

Serving Size: 1
Amount per serving: 377 g or 13.3 oz.
Preparation time 5 minutes

INGREDIENTS:
1 banana, peeled
½ cup blueberries, frozen
1 handful spinach
½ cup water or unsweetened almond milk
1 tbsp. ground flaxseed
1 tbsp. Power Shot Greens Superfood powder
1 tbsp. Coconut Milk Powder

DIRECTIONS: Blend and enjoy!

NUTRITIONAL INFORMATION

Energy (calories): 366 kcal
Protein: 9.86 g
Fats: 16.3 g
Carbohydrates: 53.39 g
Fiber: 11.7 g

Banana Cinnamon Oatmeal

Servings: 1
Serving Size: 260g or 9.1 oz.
Preparation time: 5 minutes

INGREDIENTS:
½ cup cooked oats (80 g)
¼ cup unsweetened almond milk (or Coconut milk)
1 banana mashed (120 g)
½ tsp. vanilla extract (optional)
¼ tsp. ground cinnamon (optional)
1 tsp. coconut or nut butter (optional)

TO GARNISH: ½ tsp. pumpkin seed or sunflower seeds or hemp seeds

DIRECTIONS: Combine all the ingredients in a bowl. Mix.

NUTRITIONAL INFORMATION

Energy (calories): 563 kcal
Protein: 18.89 g
Fat: 26.39 g
Carbohydrates: 69.6 g
Fiber 20 g

Coconut Yogurt with Berries & Flax Seeds

Serving Size: 1 | Amount per serving: 300 g or 10 oz.
Preparation time: 10 mins

INGREDIENTS:
1 cup of mixed berries, raw (150 g)
2 tbsp. of flaxseeds, ground
3/4 cup coconut yogurt, (170 ml)
1 tsp. of cinnamon

DIRECTIONS: Combine flax with coconut yogurt. Stir well. Add berries, stir again and sprinkle with cinnamon before serving.

NUTRITIONAL INFORMATION

Energy (calories): 563 kcal
Protein: 18.89 g
Fat: 26.39 g
Carbohydrates: 69.6 g
Fiber 20 g

Coconut Yogurt with Bananas & Chia Seeds

Servings: 1
Serving Size: 310 g or 10.9 oz.
Preparation time: 10 mins

INGREDIENTS:
1 banana, medium (120 g)
1 ½ tbsp. chia seeds (15 g)
3/4 cup coconut milk, unsweetened (170 ml)
1 tsp. of cinnamon

DIRECTIONS: Mash the banana in a bowl. Add the chia seeds and coconut yogurt. Stir everything together and keep covered in the fridge overnight. Before serving, add cinnamon.

NUTRITIONAL INFORMATION

Energy (calories): 598 kcal
Protein: 7.99 g
Fat: 47.94 g
Carbohydrates: 45.34 g
Fiber 13.6 g

Green Strawberry Smoothie

Servings: 2

Serving Size: 500 g or 17.6 oz.

INGREDIENTS:

3 cups spinach, baby leaves, organic, raw.
2 cups strawberries raw, fresh
1 cup pineapple, diced, fresh or frozen.
1 tbsp. Power Shot Greens Superfood powder
2 tbsp. flaxseed, organic powder
1-2 cups water

DIRECTIONS: Blend and enjoy!

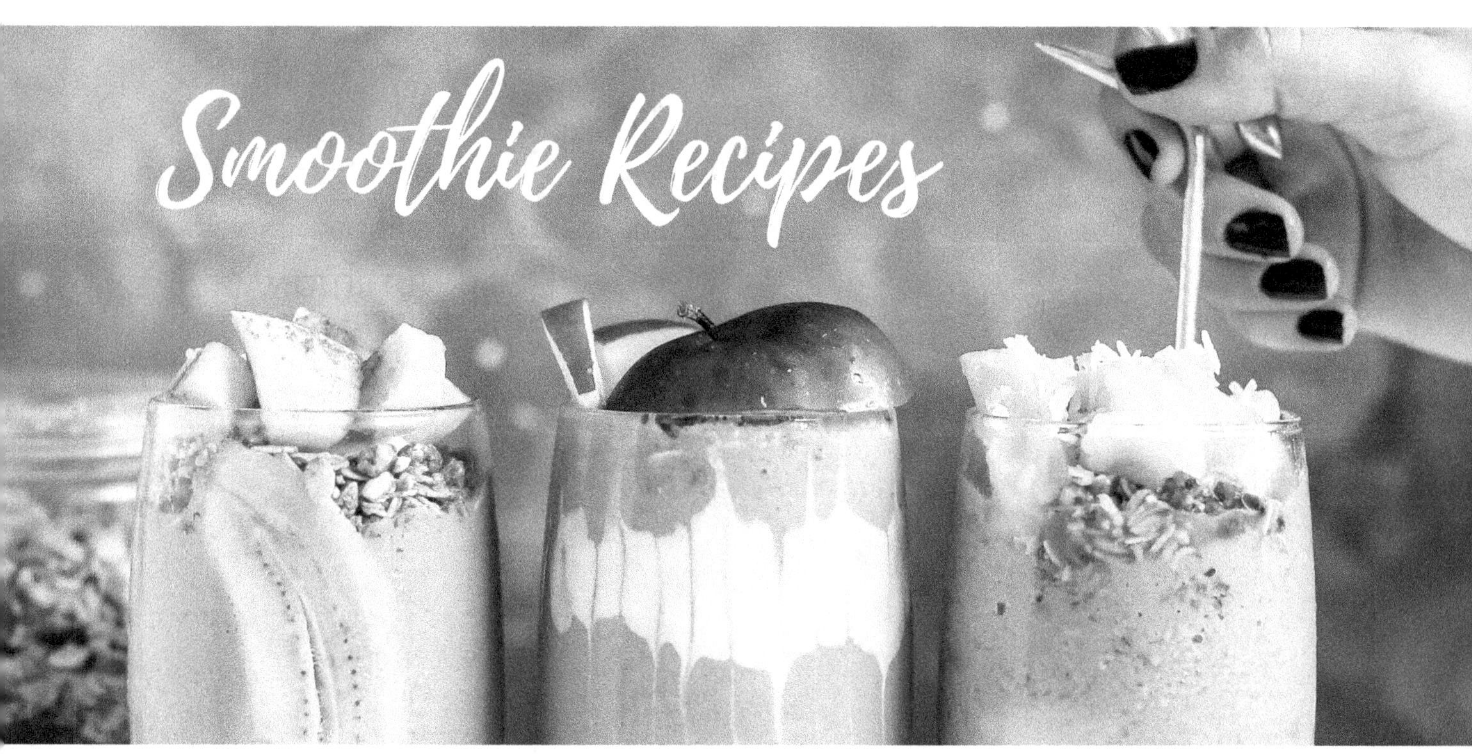

Green Apple Berry Smoothie

Servings: 2 servings (breakfast + lunch)

Amount per serving size : 450 g or 15.9 oz.

Preparation time 5 minutes

INGREDIENTS:

1 cup mixed greens
2 cups spinach, baby leaves, organic
2 cups mixed berries
1 apple, cored.
½ cup blueberries, frozen
1 tbsp. Power Shot Greens Superfood powder
2 tbsp. flaxseed, organic powder

½ to 1 cup peppermint tea

DIRECTIONS: Blend and enjoy!

Green Strawberries Smoothie

Serving size: 2 servings (breakfast + lunch)
Amount per serving: 500 g or 17.6 oz.

INGREDIENTS:

3 cups spinach, baby leaves, organic, raw
2 cups strawberries raw, fresh
1 cup pineapple, diced, fresh or frozen.
1 tbsp. Power Shot Greens Superfood powder
2 tbsp. flaxseed, organic powder
1-2 cups water

DIRECTIONS: Blend and enjoy!

NUTRITIONAL INFORMATION

Energy (calories): 196 kcal
Protein: 6.67 g
Fats: 5.32 g
Carbohydrates: 36.05 g
Fiber: 7.8 g

Green Pina Colada Smoothie

Servings: 2 servings (breakfast + lunch)
Amount per serving: 640 g or 22.6 oz.
Preparation time: 5 minutes

INGREDIENTS:

1 cup cucumbers, sliced.
2 cups pineapple chunks, fresh or frozen
1 grapefruit, peeled.
1 tbsp. lemon juice
2 apples, cored
1 tbsp. flaxseed, organic powder
1-2 tbsp. Chia seeds, presoaked in ½ cup of Coconut milk
1 tbsp. Power Shot Greens Superfood powder
1 cup water
1 tbsp. Coconut Milk powder

DIRECTIONS: Blend and enjoy!

NUTRITIONAL INFORMATION

Energy (calories): 445 kcal
Protein: 7.65 g
Fats: 21.9 g
Carbohydrates: 65 g
Fiber: 14.3 g

Green Mango Peach Smoothie

Serving size: 2 servings (breakfast + lunch)
Amount per serving: 300 g or 10.6 oz.
Preparation time: 5 minutes

INGREDIENTS:

1 cup Romaine lettuce
2 cups spinach, baby leaves, organic, raw
1 cup frozen mango-peach mix
½ a cup grapes, seedless
1 cup strawberries, fresh or frozen
½ a cup blueberries, fresh or frozen
1 tbsp. Power Shot Greens Superfood powder
2 tbsp. flaxseed, organic powder

DIRECTIONS: Blend and enjoy!

NUTRITIONAL INFORMATION

Energy (calories): 194 kcal
Protein: 6.64 g
Fats: 5.64 g
Carbohydrates: 35.11 g
Fiber: 8.2 g

Green Melon Smoothie

Serving size: 2 servings (breakfast + lunch)
Amount per serving: 300 g or 10 oz.

INGREDIENTS:
1 cup cucumber, sliced
1 cup melon chunks
½ cup Chia seeds, (80.5 g) presoak in ½ cup Coconut yogurt or water
2 tbsp. flaxseed, organic powder
1 tbsp. Power Shot Greens Superfood powder
1 tsp. mint

DIRECTIONS: Blend and enjoy!

NUTRITIONAL INFORMATION

Energy (calories): 344 kcal
Protein: 14.99 g
Fats: 20.32 g
Carbohydrates: 30.32 g
Fiber: 18.3 g

Green Honeydew Smoothie

Serving Size: 2 servings (breakfast + dinner)
Amount per serving: 520 g or 18.3 oz.
Preparation time: 5 minutes

INGREDIENTS:
2 cups Romaine lettuce
1 cup spinach, baby leaves.
2 apples, peeled, cored, chopped coarsely
1 cup honeydew chunks, fresh or frozen
2 tbsp. flaxseed, organic powder
1 tbsp. Power Shot Greens Superfood powder
1-2 cups of water

DIRECTIONS: Blend and enjoy!

NUTRITIONAL INFORMATION

Energy (calories): 203 kcal
Protein: 5.85 g
Fats: 5.25 g
Carbohydrates: 39.08 g
Fiber: 9.3 g

Green Mango Kale Smoothie

Serving Size: 2 servings
Amount per serving: 450 g 16 oz.

INGREDIENTS:
½ cup kale, baby leaves.
2 cups spinach, baby leaves, organic.
1 cup pineapple chunks, fresh or frozen
1 cup mango chunks, fresh or frozen
1 cup mixed berries, fresh or frozen.
½ cup Chia seeds, presoak in ½ a cup Coconut yogurt or water
1 tbsp. Power Shot Greens Superfood powder
2 tbsp. flaxseed, organic powder
½ to 1 cup water

DIRECTIONS: Blend and enjoy!

NUTRITIONAL INFORMATION

Energy (calories): 412 kcal
Protein: 13.45 g
Fats: 18.16 g
Carbohydrates: 57.36 g
Fiber: 22.8 g

Green Probiotics Smoothie

Serving size: 1
Amount per serving:
420 g or 14.8 oz.
Preparation time: 5 minutes

INGREDIENTS:
½ cup fresh green grapes
(80 g)
½ cup cucumber,
chopped (60 g)
½ cup pineapple, frozen
chunks (125 g)
¼ cup coconut yogurt
1 tbsp. ground flaxseed
1 tbsp. Power Shot Greens
Superfood powder
1 pinch of vanilla powder
½ cup water or unsweetened
almond milk

DIRECTIONS: Blend and
enjoy!

NUTRITIONAL INFORMATION

Energy (calories): 236 kcal
Protein: 8.18 g
Fats: 6.57 g
Carbohydrates: 40.7 g
Fiber: 6.5 g

Green Bliss Smoothie

Serving size: 1
Amount per serving:
324 g or 11.4 oz.
Preparation time: 5 minutes

INGREDIENTS:
½ cup fresh green seedless
grapes (80 g)
½ cup frozen mango chunks
(85 g)
1 handful fresh spinach or
mixed greens
1 tbsp. Power Shot Greens
Superfood powder
1 tbsp. ground flaxseed
½ cup water

DIRECTIONS: Blend and
enjoy!

NUTRITIONAL INFORMATION

Energy (calories): 236 kcal
Protein: 8.18 g
Fats: 6.57 g
Carbohydrates: 40.7 g
Fiber: 6.5 g

Green Cantaloupe Berry Smoothie

Serving size: 2 servings
(breakfast + lunch)
Amount per serving:
450 g or 15.9 oz.
Preparation time: 5 minutes

INGREDIENTS:
1 cup mixed greens
2 cups spinach,
baby leaves, organic
2 cups mixed berries (300 g)
½ cup cantaloupe
chunks (80 g)
½ cup blueberries, frozen
1 tbsp. Power Shot Greens
Superfood powder
2 tbsp. flaxseed,
organic powder
½ to 1 cup of water

DIRECTIONS: Blend and
enjoy!

NUTRITIONAL INFORMATION

Energy (calories): 217 kcal
Protein: 7.32 g
Fats: 6.07 g
Carbohydrates: 39.92 g
Fiber: 16.6 g

Green Banana Coconut Smoothie

Serving size: 1 serving
Serving Size: 377 g or 13.3 oz.
Preparation time: 5 minutes

INGREDIENTS:
1 banana, peeled
½ cup blueberries, frozen
1 handful spinach
½ cup water or unsweetened almond milk
1 tbsp. ground flaxseed
1 tbsp. Power Shot Greens Superfood powder
1 tbsp. Coconut Milk Powder

DIRECTIONS: Blend and enjoy!

NUTRITIONAL INFORMATION

Energy (calories): 366 kcal
Protein: 9.86 g
Fats: 16.3 g
Carbohydrates: 53.39 g
Fiber: 11.7 g

Green Kiwi Berry Smoothie

Servings: 1
Serving Size: 590 g or 20.8 oz.
Preparation Time: 5 minutes

INGREDIENTS:
1 small apple, cored
½ cup frozen blueberries
½ cup frozen cantaloupe chunks
1 handful spinach or arugula
1 fresh kiwi fruit, peeled
1 tbsp. ground flaxseed
1 tbsp. Power Shot Greens Superfood powder
1 tbsp. Coconut Milk Powder
½ cup water

DIRECTIONS: Blend and enjoy!

NUTRITIONAL INFORMATION

Energy (calories): 299 kcal
Protein: 9.14 g
Fats: 9.6 g
Carbohydrates: 52.82 g
Fiber: 10.3 g

Green Berry Cucumber Smoothie

Servings: 1
Serving Size: 400 g or 14.1 oz.
Preparation Time: 5 minutes

INGREDIENTS:
½ cup frozen strawberries (130 g)
½ cup frozen blueberries (80 g)
½ cup fresh cucumber, chopped
1 tbsp. ground flaxseed
1 tbsp. Power Shot Greens Superfood powder
1 tbsp. Coconut Milk Powder
½ cup water

DIRECTIONS: Blend and enjoy!

NUTRITIONAL INFORMATION

Energy (calories): 195 kcal
Protein: 7.4 g
Fats: 9.17 g
Carbohydrates: 26.28 g
Fiber: 8.2 g

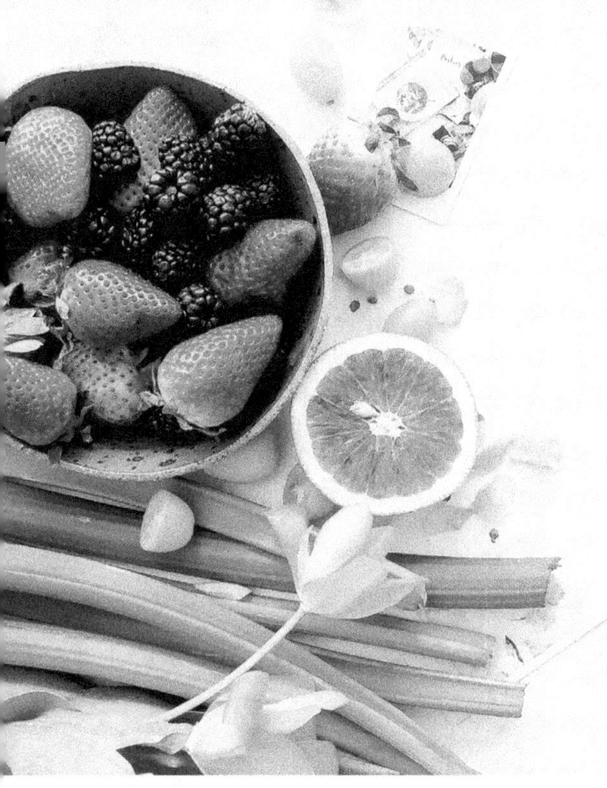

Entrees

Vegan Chilli

Servings: 6
Serving Size: 400 g or 14 oz.
Preparation Time: 10
Cooking Time: 30 minutes

INGREDIENTS:

2 tbsp. olive oil
1 medium red onion, chopped
1 large red bell pepper, chopped
2 medium carrots, chopped
2 ribs celery, chopped
½ tsp. salt, divided
4 cloves garlic, pressed or minced
2 tbsp. chili powder
2 tsp. ground cumin
1 ½ tsp. Smoked paprika
1 tsp. dried oregano
1 large can diced tomatoes
2 cans black beans
1 can of pinto beans
2 cups vegetable broth or water
1 bay leaf
2 tbsp. chopped fresh cilantro, plus more for garnishing
1 to 2 tsp. sherry vinegar
½ -1 cup of vegan ground meat (optional)

NUTRITIONAL INFORMATION

Energy (calories): 193 kcal
Protein: 7.17 g
Fats: 7.39 g
Carbohydrates: 28.24 g
Fiber: 9 g

DIRECTIONS: In a Dutch oven, warm the oil. Add chopped onion, bell pepper, carrot, celery, and salt. Cook until tender for about 10 minutes. Add garlic, chili, cumin, paprika, and oregano. Cook for a minute. Then add diced tomato with juice, beans, broth, and bay leaf, vegan ground meat and simmer for 10 minutes. For a better texture, blend the mixture in a blender until smooth.

Mediterranean Grilled Veggie Wrap

Servings: 1
Serving Size: 250 g or 8.8 oz.
Prep Time: 5 minutes

INGREDIENTS:
2 large lettuce leaves
1 tbsp. hummus
2 eggplant slices, roasted
2 slices red onion
1 zucchini slice
1 roasted red pepper slices
Garnish with sprouts or arugula or basil leaves or parsley.

DIRECTIONS: Spread 1 tbsp. hummus on lettuce leaves, layer the veggies, season and garnish, roll up as you would a burrito. Enjoy.

NUTRITIONAL INFORMATION

Energy (calories): 213 kcal

Protein: 2.99 g

Fats: 1.77 g

Carbohydrates: 19.04 g

Fiber: 4.7 g

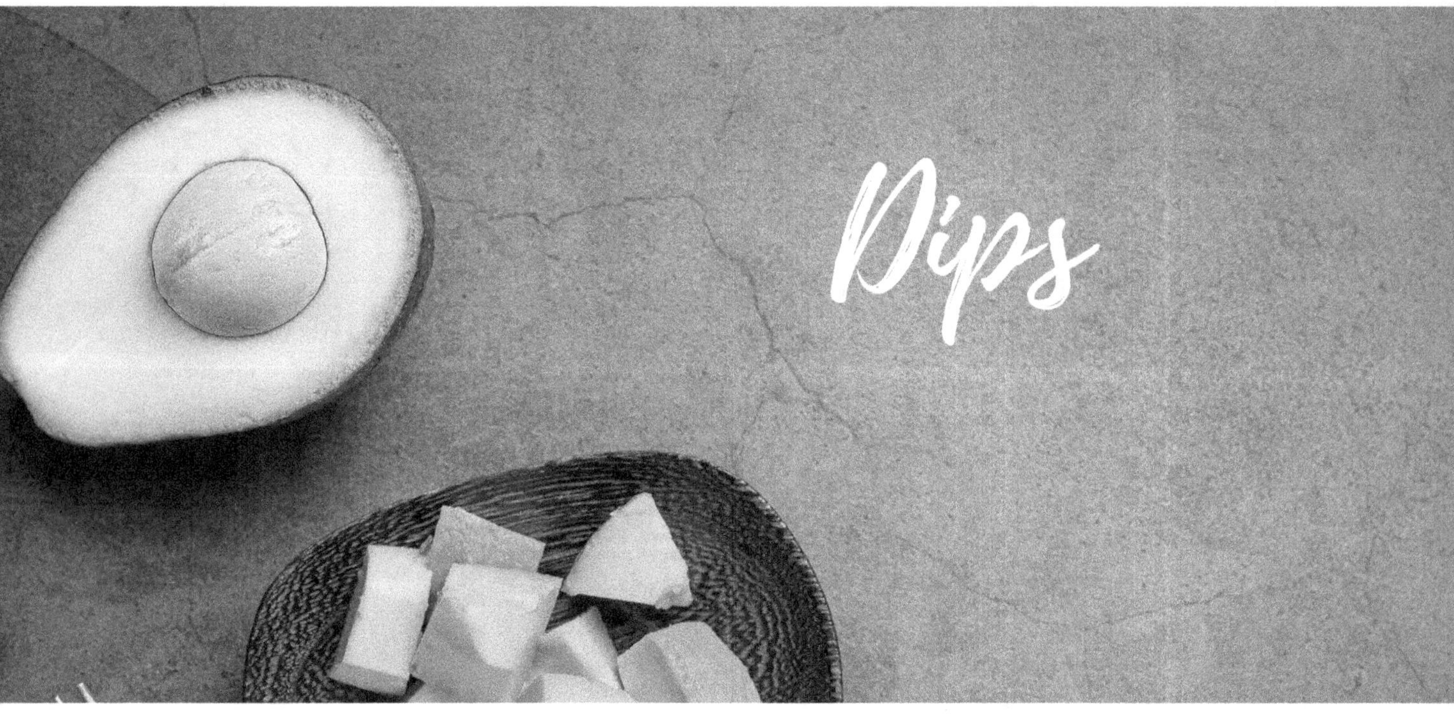

Avocado Dip

Servings: 2
Amount per serving: 100g
Prep Time: 2 minutes

INGREDIENTS:
1 avocado
4 tbsp. coconut yogurt (60 g)
½ of lime juice
¼ tsp. garlic powder
Salt to taste

DIRECTIONS: Peel, pit and mash avocado. Mix in coconut yogurt, lime juice, garlic powder, and salt. Adjust to taste.

NUTRITIONAL INFORMATION

Energy (calories): 230 kcal

Protein: 2.72 g

Fat: 20.99 g

Carbohydrates: 12.68 g

Fiber 6.9 g

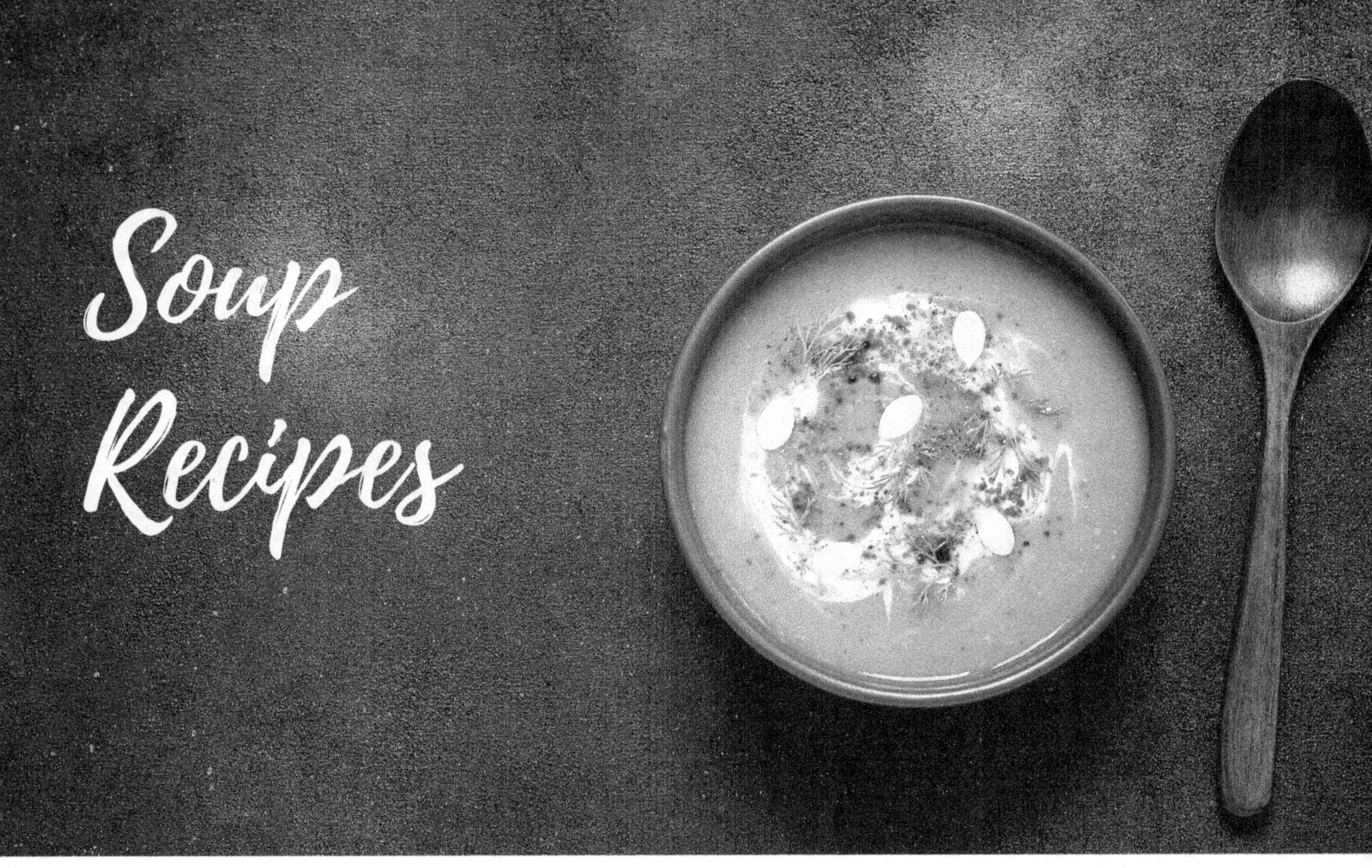

Soup Recipes

Turkey Veggie Meatball Soup

Servings: 2
Serving Size: 560 g or 19.7 oz.
Prep Time: 10 minutes
Cooking Time: 35 minutes

INGREDIENTS:
Olive oil spray
½ cup sliced celery (50 g)
¼ cup chopped onion
1 garlic clove, crushed
1 sprig fresh thyme

4 ounces lean ground turkey breast
1 cup chopped broccoli (40 g)
1 cup shredded cabbage (70 g)
3 cups low-sodium vegetable broth
1 tablespoon roughly chopped fresh parsley
1 cup chopped Swiss chard (36 g)

NUTRITIONAL INFORMATION
Energy (calories): 246 kcal
Protein: 16.94 g
Fat: 6.74 g
Carbohydrates: 30.53 g
Fiber 6.8 g

DIRECTIONS: Coat a medium saucepan with olive oil spray and heat over medium-high heat. Add the celery and onion and cook for 6 minutes. Stir in the garlic and thyme. Form the turkey into little meatballs and add to the pan. Cook the meatballs for 5 to 7 minutes, until browned, turning occasionally. Add the broccoli, cabbage, and broth. Simmer for 20 minutes. Turn off the heat, stir in the parsley and Swiss chard, and remove the thyme sprig.

Lemon Chicken Soup

Servings: 2-4
Serving Size: 560 g or 19.7 oz.
Prep Time: 10 minutes
Cooking time: 50 minutes

INGREDIENTS:
2 bone-in chicken thighs (300 g)
1 onion, chopped
2 celery sticks, chopped
1 medium carrot, chopped
2 medium potatoes, peeled, chopped (430g)
4 cups water or chicken broth
1 green bell pepper, seeded and chopped
1 small tomato, chopped
1 tbsp. salt
1 tbsp. olive oil
fresh ground black pepper to taste
1 tbsp. Italian spice mix
1 tbsp. basil
¼ cup of rice, uncooked (46 g)
Juice of 1 lemon and lemon zest

TO GARNISH: Fresh chopped scallion and Italian parsley or dill.

NUTRITIONAL INFORMATION

Energy (calories): 402 kcal
Protein: 24.35 g
Fat: 10.97 g
Carbohydrates: 52.54 g
Fiber 6.9 g

DIRECTIONS: In a large pot, place chicken in the water (or broth) with salt and ½ of the onion and celery. Bring it to boil. Reduce heat, cover and simmer for 30 minutes. Remove the chicken from the pot with thongs. Add all the rest of the vegetables, rice and spices and cook for 15 minutes uncovered on medium heat. Take the chicken from the bone, discard skin and bones. Put chicken pieces in the soup. Add lemon juice and zest. Serve.

Green Power Soup

Servings: 8 serving
Serving size: 380 g 13.4oz
Preparation Time: 30 minutes
Cooking Time: 10 min.

INGREDIENTS:
1 onion, rough chopped
½ head of garlic, rough chopped ~3 cloves
½" ginger, rough chopped
8 cups vegetable stock or water
1 cup cauliflower, optional
1 cup broccoli
2 small leeks
½ bunch kale ~4 cups, chopped
4 cups spinach, fresh or frozen
Juice of half a lemon

NUTRITIONAL INFORMATION

Energy (calories): 131 kcal
Protein: 5.21 g
Fats: 2.49 g
Carbohydrates: 24.01 g
Fiber: 3.6 g

DIRECTIONS: Begin by cooking the onion in water, then add the ginger and garlic and cook until soft. Keep on eye on the water because if it gets too low then things might burn. Now, add the water or vegetable stock, cauliflower, broccoli, and leeks. Bring these to a boil and then turn it down to simmer for 10 minutes. The vegetables should be tender when done. Now, add the kale and spinach and allow to simmer for another 4 minutes or until these are soft. Blend all the ingredients together and enjoy the goodness.

Lentil Soup with Greens

Servings: 1
Serving Size: 380 g or 13.4 oz.
Preparation Time: 10 minutes
Cooking time: 20 minutes

INGREDIENTS:

1 tbsp. oil
1 clove garlic minced
1 small onion
1 large carrot (thinly sliced)
1 stalk celery (thinly sliced)
1/8 tsp. salt and black pepper (divided/plus more to taste)
1 cup vegetable broth (plus more as needed)
1 tbsp. of fresh rosemary or thyme
¼ cup of uncooked green or brown lentils (thoroughly rinsed and drained)
½ cup of chopped kale or collard greens
1 tsp. paprika
1 small cam diced tomato (optional)
pinch cayenne pepper

NUTRITIONAL INFORMATION

Energy (calories): 125 kcal
Protein: 3.68 g
Fats: 5 g
Carbohydrates: 19.17 g
Fiber: 4.1 g

DIRECTIONS: Heat a pot over medium heat. Once hot, add oil, garlic, shallots, carrot, and celery. Season with a bit of salt and pepper and stir again. Sauté for 4-5 minutes or until veggies slightly tender and get golden brown. Be careful not to burn the garlic (turn heat down if it's cooking too quickly.) Add vegetable broth and (diced tomato) rosemary or thyme and increase heat to medium high. Bring to a rolling simmer. Then add lentils and stir. Once simmering again, reduce heat to low and simmer uncovered for 15-20 minutes or until lentils are tender. Add your greens, stir, and cover. Cook for 3-4 minutes more to wilt. Then taste and adjust flavor as needed, adding more salt and pepper for overall flavor, vegetable broth if it's become too thick, or herbs for earthy flavor.

Hippocrates Healing Soup

Servings: 6 servings
Serving size: 250 g or 8.8 oz.
Preparation Time: 15 minutes
Cooking Time: 1.5 -2 hr.

INGREDIENTS:

1 medium celery root, or 3-4 celery branches
2 small or 1 large leek
2 medium onions
1 tbsp. of parsley
1-1 ½ pounds of tomatoes
1 pound potatoes
Garlic to taste (may also be squeezed raw into the hot soup, instead of cooking it)

NUTRITIONAL INFORMATION

Energy (calories): 110 kcal
Protein: 3.3 g
Fats: 0.4 g
Carbohydrates: 24.91 g
Fiber: 4.1 g

DIRECTIONS: Begin by washing and scrubbing your vegetables thoroughly and coarsely chopping them. The size of the chop isn't going to matter much because you're just going to puree this soup in the end. Now, in a large pot, add enough water to just cover the vegetables and bring to a boil. Note that there is no need to use broth or stock in this recipe because the end result is going to be flavorful on its own. You want to simmer the soup at low heat for 1.5 to 2 hours, or until the vegetables are soft. If you're really in a hurry you can do 1 hour, but it's much better when you take the time to do it right. Now, blend the ingredients really well and remove any fibers. You can serve it right away or store in the refrigerator for up to 2 days.

Cabbage Detox Soup

Servings: 4-6 servings
Amount per serving 730 g –
488 g or 25.7 oz. to 17.2oz
Prep Time: 10 minutes
Cook Time: 20 minutes

INGREDIENTS:

6 cups veggie broth
2 onions, sliced or chopped
4 cloves garlic, minced
2 carrots, medium, peeled, diced
1 green, yellow, red, bell pepper, diced
1 cup celery, diced
1/2 head of cabbage, chopped (620 g)
1 tsp. lemon juice
1 tsp. organic apple cider vinegar
1 cup V8 vegetable juice
2-3 medium fresh tomatoes, diced
6 large fresh scallions, chopped
¼ tsp. black pepper
1 cup fresh spinach or kale or bok choy
1 tsp. oregano
1 tsp. basil
¼ tsp. salt
2 bay leaves
¼ tsp. fresh parsley or cilantro, chopped
2 tbsp. sunflower or grape seed oil
pinch of cayenne pepper (optional)

NUTRITIONAL INFORMATION

Energy (calories): 234 kcal

Protein: 8.34 g

Fats: 5.88 g

Carbohydrates: 41.2 g

Fiber: 7.4 g

DIRECTIONS: Bring veggie broth to a boil in a pot. Add all the ingredients except the scallions and spinach. Reduce heat to simmer. Cook until vegetables are tender, about 15 minutes. Add the spinach and cook for 3-5 min. Taste broth and adjust seasoning if needed. Garnish with ¼ tsp. fresh parsley or cilantro. Serve and enjoy!

Bean Soup

Servings: 1
Serving size: 550 g or 19.4 oz.
Preparation time 5 minute
Cooking time: 25 minutes

INGREDIENTS:

1 tbsp. olive oil
1 small onion, chopped
1 garlic clove, minced
1 small carrot, chopped
1 celery rib, chopped
1 cup vegetable broth
1/4 tsp. dried thyme
1/8 tsp. oregano
Salt and pepper to taste
4 oz. canned black beans drained and rinsed
2 cups baby spinach
Fresh parsley for serving

NUTRITIONAL INFORMATION

Energy (calories): 332 kcal

Protein: 11.98 g

Fat: 15.01 g

Carbohydrates: 41.04 g

Fiber 15.1 g

DIRECTIONS: Heat olive on medium high heat in a pot. Add onion and garlic and cook until onions are translucent, about 3-5 minutes. Add carrot, celery, and cook for an additional 2-3 minutes. Add vegetable broth and beans, and bring to a boil, reduce heat and simmer for 15 minutes. Stir in the spinach and thyme, oregano, salt and pepper, and continue simmering until the spinach wilts, about 2 minutes. Remove from the heat, sprinkle fresh parsley and serve with cucumber dill salad.

Thai Curry Zucchini Soup

Servings: 2 servings
Amount per serving: 460 g or 16.2 oz.
Preparation time: 5 minutes
Cooking time: 20 minutes

INGREDIENTS:

1 tbsp. coconut oil or olive oil
1 lb. zucchini, cut into small ½-inch pieces
1 medium yellow onion, chopped
2 garlic cloves, pressed or chopped
2 tbsp. Thai Curry Paste
1 tsp. ground coriander
¼ tsp. ground cumin
1/8 tsp. salt
1 tbsp. fresh lime juice
2 cups vegetable broth (16 oz.)
¼ a cup full fat coconut milk for drizzling on top
¼ cup large, unsweetened shredded coconut flakes
Handful fresh cilantro leaves, chopped

NUTRITIONAL INFORMATION

Energy (calories): 125 kcal
Protein: 3.68 g
Fats: 5 g
Carbohydrates: 19.17 g
Fiber: 4.1 g

DIRECTIONS: Heat oil in a pot over medium heat. Once the oil is shimmering, add chopped veggies and spices. Stir to combine. Cook, stirring occasionally, until veggies softens, about 3 to 5 minutes. Add broth. Bring the mixture to a boil, then reduce heat and simmer for next 15 to 20 minutes. Toast the coconut flakes in a medium skillet over medium-low heat, stirring frequently, until fragrant and golden on the edges. Keep an eye on them so they don't burn. Transfer coconut flakes to a bowl to cool. Remove the soup from heat and let it cool slightly. Transfer the contents to a blender and purée the mixture until smooth. Stir the lime juice into the blended soup. Ladle half amount of soup into bowl. Use a spoon to drizzle coconut milk over it. Top the soup with toasted coconut flakes and a sprinkle of chopped fresh cilantro.

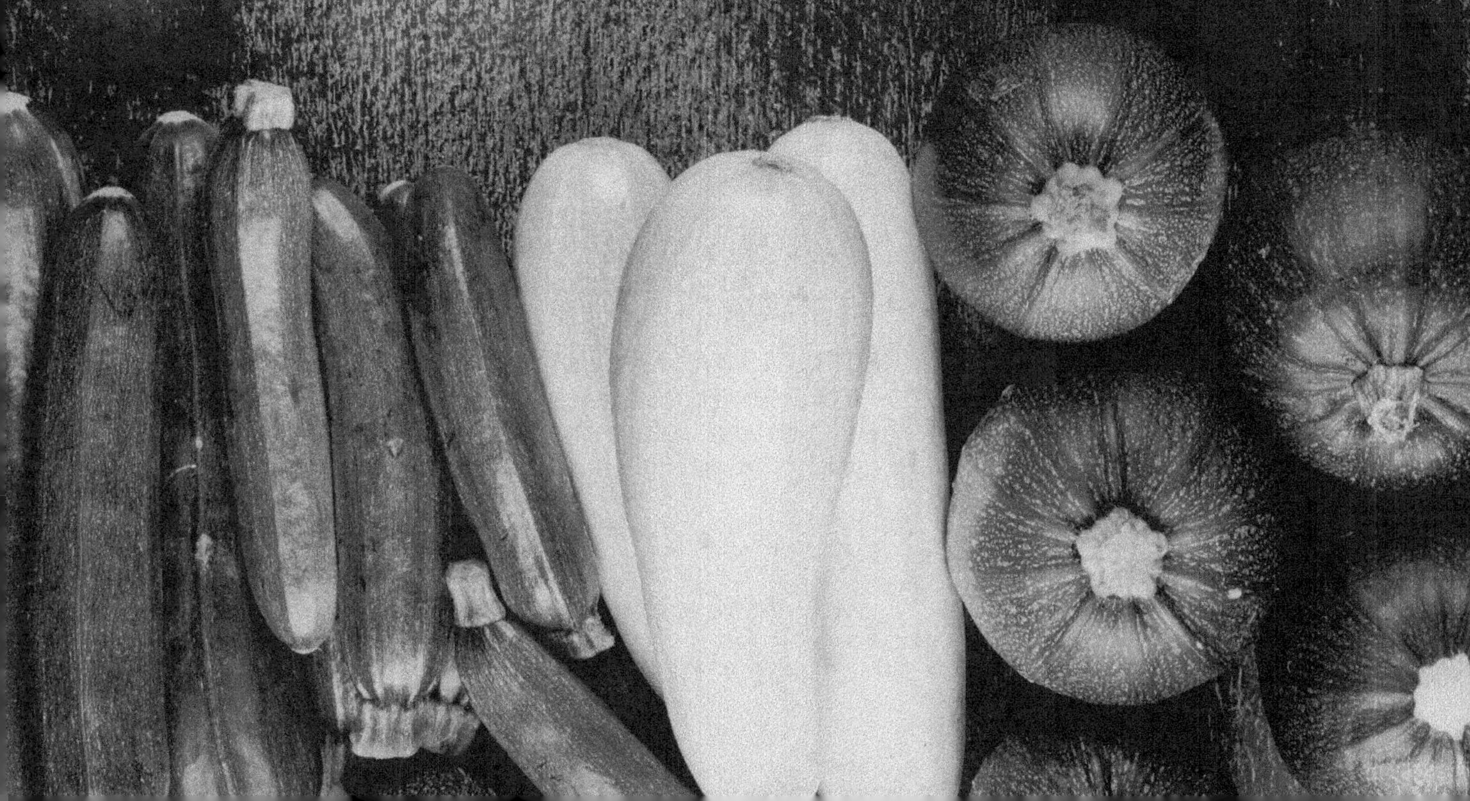

Salads and Sides

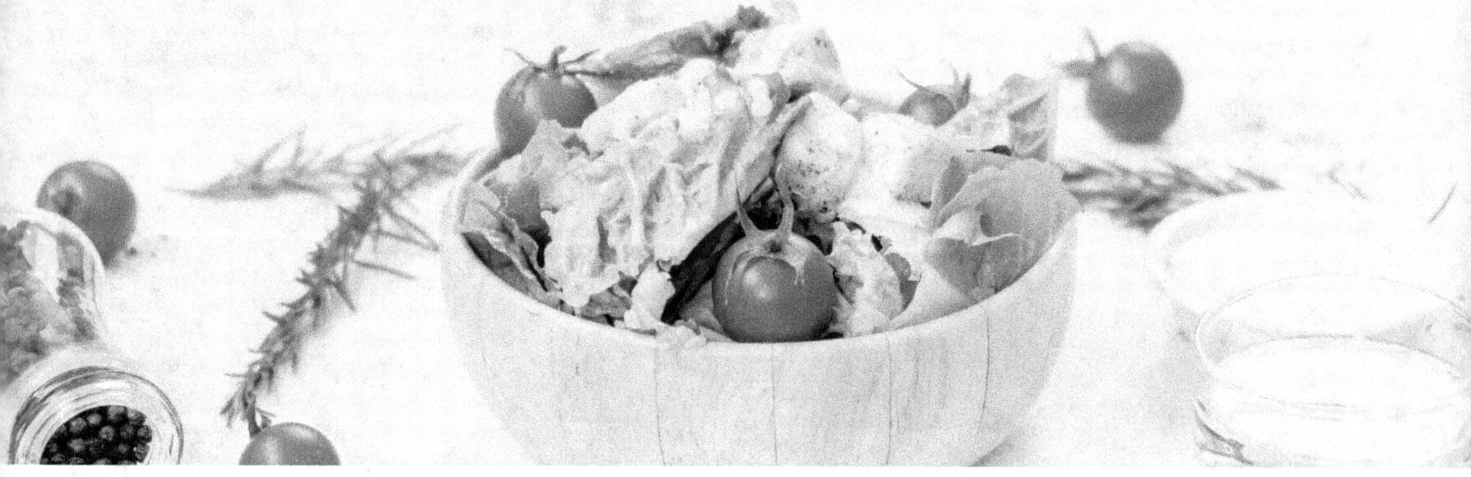

Raw Beet Salad with Seeds

INGREDIENTS:

1 small raw beet, peeled and grated (80 g)
½ juice lemon

1 tbsp. flax oil
2 tbsp. roasted sunflower seeds

> **NUTRITIONAL INFORMATION**
> Energy (calories): 263 kcal,
> Protein: 3.64 g
> Fat: 22.8 g
> Carbohydrates: 13 g
> Fibers: 3.9 g

Grilled Veggies

Servings: 2
Serving size: 520 g or 18.3 oz.
Prep Time: 10 minutes
Cooking Time: 15 minutes

INGREDIENTS:

1 medium eggplant, sliced in 1/4 inch planks (460 g)
2 roasted red pepper, sliced into strips
1 medium zucchini, sliced into wheels (200 g)
3 garlic gloves, whole
1 medium onion, quartered
sprouts to garnish

salt, pepper, Italian spice mix, paprika to taste
TO GARNISH: fresh basil leaves, scallions, sesame seeds.

DIRECTIONS: Preheat oven to 375 F. Brush all the veggies with olive oil, add salt, pepper, Italian spice mix, and paprika on each. Bake for 15 minutes. *Note: Leftover grilled veggies can be used for Grilled Veggie wrap, or Poke bowl.*

> **NUTRITIONAL INFORMATION**
> Energy (calories): 117 kcal
> Protein: 4.4 g
> Fat: 0.74 g
> Carbohydrates: 27.37 g
> Fiber: 10.2g

Greek Salad

Servings: 2
Amount per serving: 350 g
Prep Time: 10 minutes

INGREDIENTS:
1 cucumber, sliced (200 g)
2 scallions, chopped (30 g)
2 medium ripe tomatoes (245 g)
1 green bell pepper, seeded and chopped (120 g)
2 oz. pitted Kalamata olives
1 tbsp. olive oil
Salt and pepper to taste
small amount of fresh dill, chopped
Garnish: chopped parsley

DIRECTIONS: Add all the ingredients in a bowl and toss gently. Garnish with parsley.

NUTRITIONAL INFORMATION

Energy (calories): 161 kcal
Protein: 3.24 g
Fat: 11.69 g
Carbohydrates: 14.11 g
Fiber 4.9 g

Green Salad

Servings: 2
Serving size: 85 g or 3 oz.
Prep Time: 10 minutes

INGREDIENTS:
1 cup Romaine lettuce, shredded (50 g)
5 radishes, sliced (25 g)
½ cucumber, sliced (100 g)
2 scallions, chopped
Salt and pepper to taste
small amount of fresh dill, chopped

DRESSING:
1 tsp. Apple cider vinegar
1 tbsp. olive oil

DIRECTIONS: Add all the ingredients in a bowl and mix thoroughly.

NUTRITIONAL INFORMATION

Energy (calories): 83 kcal
Protein: 1.27 g
Fat: 7.06 g
Carbohydrates: 5.03 g
Fiber 1.6 g

Asian Salad with Sesame Ginger Dressing

Servings: 4
Serving size: 180g or 6 oz.
Preparation Time: 10 minutes

INGREDIENTS:
4 carrots, grated
1 large red pepper, finely diced
2 celery stalks, finely diced
½ medium red onion, finely diced
½ cup cilantro or parsley, chopped
4 tbsp. toasted sesame seeds
½ cup roasted peanuts, almonds, or cashews

DRESSING:
3 tbsp. of sesame oil
2 tbsp. fresh squeezed lemon juice
2 tsp. soy sauce
1 tbsp. of grated ginger
1 small clove of garlic, crushed
Sea salt to taste

DIRECTIONS: Combine all the dressing ingredients in a small bowl and whisk together. Set aside. Toss all the remaining ingredients together in a medium-sized bowl. Pour over the dressing and toss to coat.

NUTRITIONAL INFORMATION

Energy (calories): 286kcal
Protein: 7.76g
Fats: 23.9 g
Carbohydrates: 17.06 g
Fibers: 6.2g

Cucumber Dill Salad

Servings: 4   Amount per Serving: 120g or 4 oz.
Preparation Time: 5 minutes

INGREDIENTS:
2 cucumbers, sliced
1 spring onion, sliced
1/4 cup white vinegar
2 tbsp. oil
1-1/2 tsp. dried dill, or to taste
Salt and pepper to taste

DIRECTIONS: Toss together the cucumbers and onion in a large bowl. Combine oil with vinegar, and salt. Drizzle over the salad and sprinkle with fresh dill. Serve.

NUTRITIONAL INFORMATION
Energy (calories): 78kcal
Protein: 0.73g
Fats: 7.03 g
Carbohydrates: 2.81 g
Fiber: 0.9g

Cranberry Cilantro Quinoa Salad

Servings: 2
Serving size: 275 g or 9.7 oz.

INGREDIENTS:
½ cup quinoa, precooked (85 g)
1 tbsp. of dried cranberries
½ cup cucumber, chopped
3 tbsp. fresh cilantro, chopped
1/2 cup bell pepper, diced
1 roasted pepper, diced
1 tomato, chopped
1 tbsp. almonds, toasted, sliced
2 tbsp. carrots, grated/ shredded
½ lime, juice
½ lemon, juice
½ cup green chopped onion
salt and pepper to taste
olive oil for drizzling as desired
pinch of cumin or to taste (optional)
1 additional lime sliced into wedges to garnish

DIRECTIONS: Combine freshly cooked quinoa with all the vegetables and nuts. Season to taste. For best results, chill salad before serving. Enjoy!

NUTRITIONAL INFORMATION
Energy (calories): 264 kcal
Protein: 9.36 g
Fats: 6.69 g
Carbohydrates: 44.33 g
Fiber: 7.25 g

Mushroom Gravy

Servings: 2
Serving size: 180 g
Prep Time: 10 minutes

INGREDIENTS:
1 cup sliced mushrooms (70 g)
1 cup almond milk
1 tbsp. vegan butter
salt and pepper
garlic powder
onion powder
2 oz. cornstarch
Italian spice mix
pinch of nutmeg (optional)

NUTRITIONAL INFORMATION
Energy (calories): 207 kcal
Protein: 4.25 g
Fat: 6.84 g
Carbohydrates: 32.08 g
Fiber 1.1 g

DIRECTIONS: Wash mushrooms and place in pot with vegan butter. Put top on and cook on medium heat until softened. The juice of the mushroom will release and mushrooms will shrink. Add nut milk and spices. Stir gently for a few minutes. To thicken, mix cornstarch with a small amount of water and add to mushrooms. Mix until it thickens. Remove from heat. Pour over chickpea meatloaf.

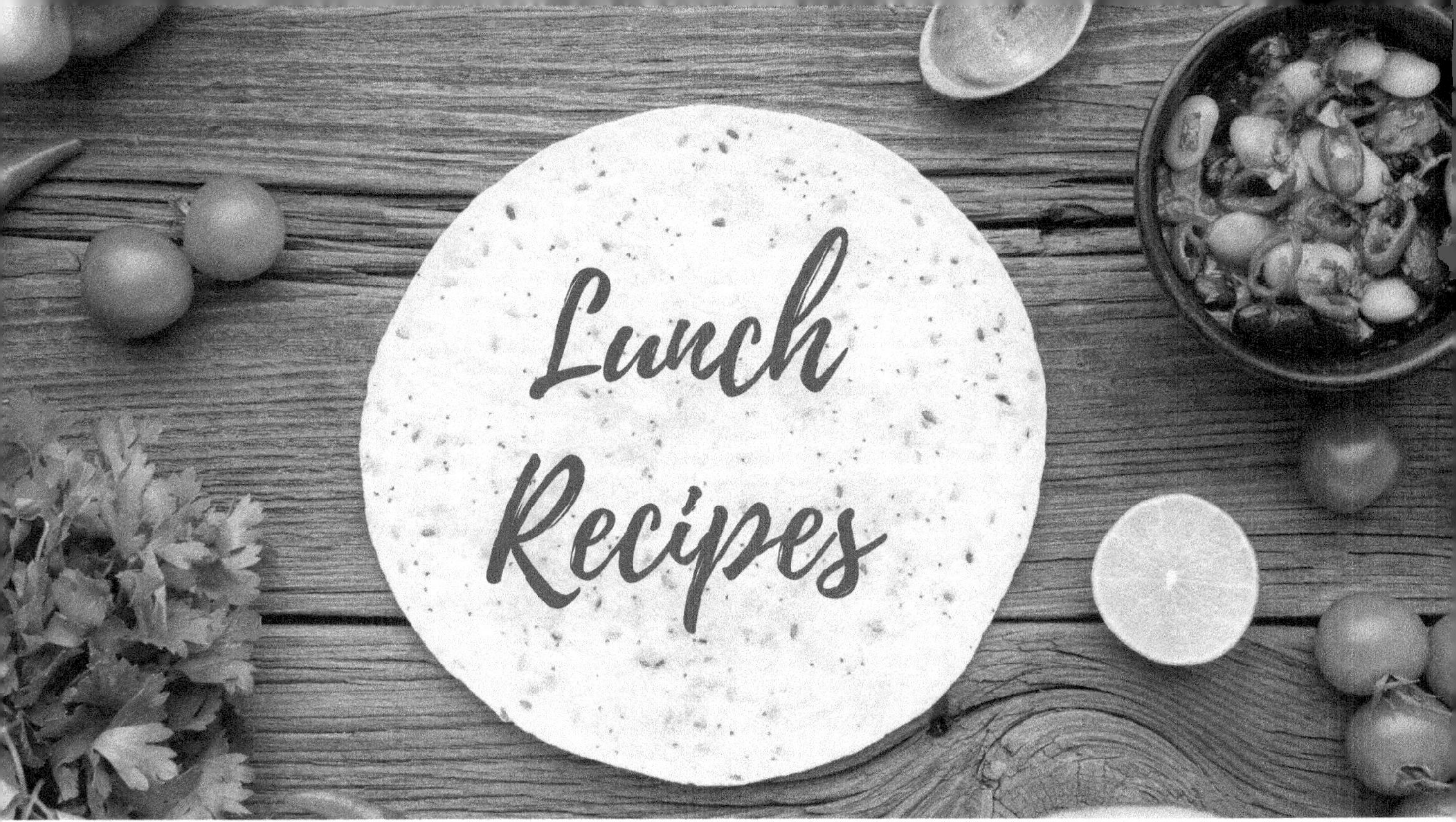

Seaweed Congee "Chinese Rice Porridge"

Servings: 5
Serving size: 410 g
Preparation Time: 15 minutes
Cooking Time: 10 minutes

INGREDIENTS:
½ cup short grain rice (100 g)
1 inch piece fresh ginger, minced
2 cloves garlic, minced
7 dried shiitake mushrooms, soaked in hot water, chopped
5 cups water
½ small head Bok Choy, chopped
2-6" strips of dried Kombu
FOR TOPPINGS:
USE ANY ONE OR MORE
5 oz. of crispy tofu cubes
1 medium carrot, finely chopped
2 tbsp. scallions
2 tbsp. cashews or pumpkin seeds, toasted
1 green onion, sliced
Chili oil, etc.
Salt to taste

DIRECTIONS: In a pot, place water and rice over medium heat. Add mushrooms, ginger, garlic, Kombu and salt (or Dulse) to the pot. Stir and close the lid. Cook until rice is done, about 30 minutes. Stir a couple of times while it is cooking. Add Bok Choy and simmer for 10 minutes. Ladle into bowls. Serve with toppings.

NUTRITIONAL INFORMATION
Energy (calories): 163 kcal
Protein: 8.58 g
Fat: 4.31 g
Carbohydrates: 24.89 g
Fiber 3.3 g

Lettuce Taco Chicken Wrap

Servings: 1
Serving Size: 373 g or 13 oz.
Preparation Time: 10 minutes
Cooking Time: 20 minutes

INGREDIENTS:
4 oz. cooked chicken breast, chopped
1 lemon (juice)
1/8 tsp. kosher salt
Fresh ground pepper
¼ tsp. paprika
2 oz. Pico de Gallo
1 avocado, chopped
Handful shredded lettuce
2 large lettuce leaves
Garnish with fresh cilantro

DIRECTIONS: In each lettuce leaf, layer the shredded lettuce, Pico de Gallo, Avocado, cilantro and seasonings. Wrap the lettuce leaves around the filling and serve.

NUTRITIONAL INFORMATION

Energy (calories): 568 kcal
Protein: 41.38 g
Fats: 33.97 g
Carbohydrates: 32.51 g
Fiber: 15.5 g

Rice Tortilla Wrap with Veggies

Serving Size: 1
Serving Size: 300 g or 10.6 oz.
Preparation time: 5 minutes
Cooking time 15 minutes

INGREDIENTS:
1 large rice tortilla (homemade)
6 asparagus spears, grilled
1 cup shredded lettuce
1 small cucumber, cut into strips
1 cup of arugula

INGREDIENTS FOR RICE TORTILLA:
1 cup water
1 cup Rice-Flour
pinch salt

DIRECTIONS: Bring water to a boil, add a bit of salt and rice flour. Stir the mass with wooden spoon to combine. Let it cool a bit to form dough. Pour the batter on wide surface. Pour a bit of water and wet your hands too. Knead the dough, using a bit more water. It takes around 10 minutes to prepare good dough. Split the dough into 8 crack free balls (use more water if needed). Using a rolling pin flatten it in a circle shape with desired thickness. You can flatten the balls using tortilla press too. Put some oil on both sides of the tortilla press, before flattening them. Heat the skillet to medium high heat. Place the tortilla and cook for a minute, flip it and cook for another minute on the other side. If it starts to fluff use a paper towel to press it down. Keep the rest of tortilla in air tight container. Don't freeze them, since they will become hard and break. Fill tortilla with grilled asparagus and fresh veggies. Serve.

NUTRITIONAL INFORMATION

Energy (calories): 213 kcal
Protein: 6.38 g
Fats: 7.79 g
Carbohydrates: 30.24 g
Fiber: 3.6 g

Green Bean Stew

Serving Size: 1
Amount per serving: 450 g or 8 oz.
Preparation time :5 minutes
Cooking time: 25-30 minutes

INGREDIENTS:
8 oz. green beans
1 carrot, sliced
¼ tsp ground coriander seeds
2 tbsp. virgin olive oil
1 small onion, chopped
1 tomato, peeled and pureed
½ cup parsley, chopped
2 smaller size potatoes, quartered or in thick slices
Salt and pepper to taste
1 - 1½ cups of water

DIRECTIONS: Heat oil in a pot; add green beans, coriander, pepper, and carrot. Stir gently for about 3-4 minutes.
Add the onion and continue cooking and stirring until it becomes translucent (about 2-3 minutes). Add salt, sliced potatoes, and tomato. Add enough water to almost cover the beans and potatoes. Bring to a boil, cover the pot and reduce heat to medium, simmer for 10 minutes, add the parsley and continue cooking until potatoes are fork-tender (about 10-15 minutes more). You might need to add a bit of water if you notice that a lot of it is gone during cooking.

NUTRITIONAL INFORMATION
Energy (calories): 576 kcal
Protein: 9.98 g
Fat: 28.89 g
Carbohydrates: 75.7 g
Fiber 13.6 g

Hawaiian Tofu Poke Salad

Servings: 1 serving
Amount per serving: 330 g or 11.6 oz.
Preparation time: 10 minutes

INGREDIENTS:
1 scallion greens, thinly sliced
1 tbsp. reduced-sodium tamari
1 tsp. toasted (dark) sesame oil
1 tsp. toasted sesame seeds
1 tsp. grated fresh ginger
3 oz. extra-firm tofu, drained and cut into ½ -inch pieces
1 cup zucchini noodles (chop with spiralizers)
2 tsp. rice vinegar
1 medium carrot, shredded
½ a cup peas (60 g)
1 tbsp. toasted chopped walnuts
1 tbsp. chopped fresh basil

DIRECTIONS: Whisk scallion greens, tamari, 1/2 tsp. of rice vinegar, oil, sesame seeds, ginger, in a medium bowl. Add tofu to the sauce in the medium bowl and gently toss to coat. Combine zucchini noodles and vinegar in a large bowl. Top with marinated tofu, sliced or chopped carrot and pea shoots, and walnuts and basil.

NUTRITIONAL INFORMATION
Energy (calories): 244 kcal
Protein: 13.45 g
Fats: 15.34 g
Carbohydrates: 17.43 g
Fiber: 4.9 g

Grilled Veggie Wrap

Servings: 1
Serving Size: 250 g or 8.8 oz.
Prep Time: 5 minutes

INGREDIENTS:
2 large lettuce leaves
1 tbsp. hummus
2 eggplant slices, roasted
2 slices of red onion
1 zucchini slice
1 roasted red pepper slices
Garnish with sprouts or arugula or basil leaves or parsley.

DIRECTIONS: Spread 1 tbsp. hummus on lettuce leaves, layer the veggies, season and garnish, roll up as you would a burrito. Enjoy.

NUTRITIONAL INFORMATION

Energy (calories): 213 kcal
Protein: 2.99 g
Fats: 1.77 g
Carbohydrates: 19.04 g
Fiber: 4.7 g

Tomato, Cauliflower & Spinach Curry

Serves: 2
Serving Size: 270 g or 9.5 oz.
Preparation Time: 10 minutes
Cooking Time: 25 minutes

INGREDIENTS:
1 onion, sliced
2 tbsp. oil, for frying
2 tbsp. curry paste,
½ tsp. ground turmeric
1 small cauliflower, cut into bite-sized florets (270 g)
3 ripe plum tomatoes, quartered
Handful spinach, roughly chopped

DIRECTIONS: Heat oil in a skillet over medium heat and add onion to sauté for 10 minutes along with salt. Stir in curry paste and turmeric. Cook for 2 minutes then add tomatoes, cauliflower, and quarter cup water and let it simmer for 15 minutes. Add spinach and cook for 3 to 5 minutes. Serve.

NUTRITIONAL INFORMATION

Energy (calories): 198 kcal
Protein: 4.81 g
Fats: 15.13 g
Carbohydrates: 15.19 g
Fiber: 7.7 g

Grilled Wild Salmon

Servings: 1 serving
Serving size: 290g or 10.2 oz.
Preparation time: 5 minutes
Cooking time: 30 minutes

INGREDIENTS:
1 tbsp. of olive oil
Salt and pepper to taste
7 oz. wild Salmon filet
2 tbsp. of basil-pesto-hummus
½ lemon, then sliced
2 cloves garlic, minced

DIRECTIONS: Preheat oven to 450 F and line a baking sheet with aluminum foil.
Season both sides of the salmon with oil, salt, pepper and garlic. Place in the middle of the sheet pan. Bake it for next 15 minutes until the salmon is done. Top the salmon with basil pesto hummus and serve with Greek salad.

NUTRITIONAL INFORMATION

Energy (calories): 477 kcal
Protein: 44.85g
Fats: 27.94 g
Carbohydrates: 9.74 g
Fibers: 1.4 g

Vegan Chickpea Meatloaf

Servings: 4
Serving Size: 160g or 5.6 oz.
Prep Time: 10 minutes
Cooking Time: 55 minutes

INGREDIENTS:

1-14 oz. cans or 1 1/2 cups cooked chickpeas, drained and rinsed
½ onion, diced
1 celery stalk, chopped
½ cup ground oatmeal (120 g)
1 carrot, diced
1 garlic clove, minced
¼ cup ground flaxseed (40 g)
¼ cup unflavored soy or almond milk
1 tbsp. vegan Worcestershire sauce
1 tbsp. soy sauce or tamari
1 tbsp. olive oil
1 tbsp. ground flax seeds
1 tbsp. tomato paste
½ tsp. liquid smoke
1/8 tsp. black pepper

NUTRITIONAL INFORMATION

Energy (calories): 246 kcal
Protein: 8.7 g
Fats: 11.13 g
Carbohydrates: 30.33 g
Fiber: 8.8 g

DIRECTIONS: Preheat oven to 375°. Lightly oil a 9 inch loaf pan and arrange a strip of parchment paper width-wise along the center, with just a bit hanging over the sides. Working in batches if needed, place all meatloaf ingredients into food processor bowl and pulse until chickpeas are broken up and ingredients are well mixed, stopping to scrape down sides of bowl as needed. Do not over blend. If working in batches, transfer each batch to a large mixing bowl when complete and then mix by hand. Press mixture into prepared loaf pan and bake 30 minutes. While meatloaf bakes, stir glaze ingredients together in a small bowl. Remove loaf from oven after 30 minutes and spoon glaze over top of loaf. Bake another 20-25 minutes. Remove from oven and allow to cool at least 10 minutes before cutting.

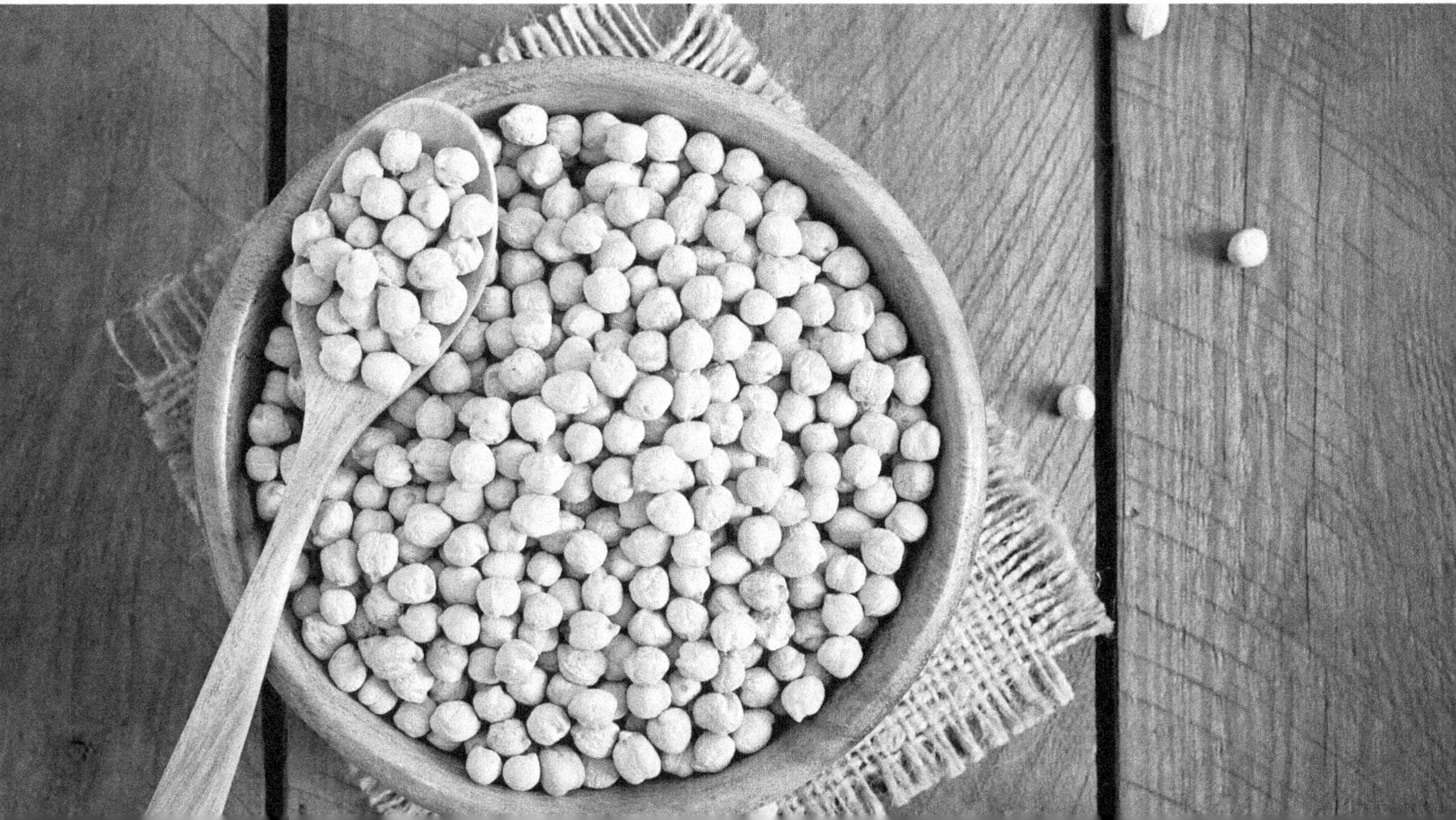

Stuffed Bell Peppers with Ground Turkey

Serving Size: 1
Amount per serving: 460g or 16.2 oz.
Preparation time: 10 minutes
Cooking time: 4 minutes

INGREDIENTS:
1 tsp. of extra-virgin olive oil
½ of leek, smaller, chopped (45 g)
1 clove garlic, minced
3 oz. 90 g of ground turkey
½ a cup of canned diced tomatoes (120 g)
1 tsp. uncooked rice
1 tsp. sesame seeds
½ tsp. dried oregano
Salt and pepper to taste
1 bell pepper top and core removed
Freshly chopped parsley, for garnish

NUTRITIONAL INFORMATION
Energy (calories): 477 kcal
Protein: 17.94 g
Fat: 32.73 g
Carbohydrates: 39.08 g
Fiber 7.4 g

DIRECTIONS: In a skillet over medium heat, heat oil. Cook onion until soft, about 5 minutes. Stir in garlic and cook until fragrant, about 1 minute more. Add ground turkey and cook, breaking up meat with a wooden spoon, then stir in rice, sesame seeds and diced tomatoes. Season it with oregano, salt, and pepper. Let simmer until liquid has reduced slightly, about next 5 minutes. Cut pepper and remove the seeds. Spoon the beef mixture into each pepper half. Microwave it for 4 minutes. Garnish with parsley before serving.

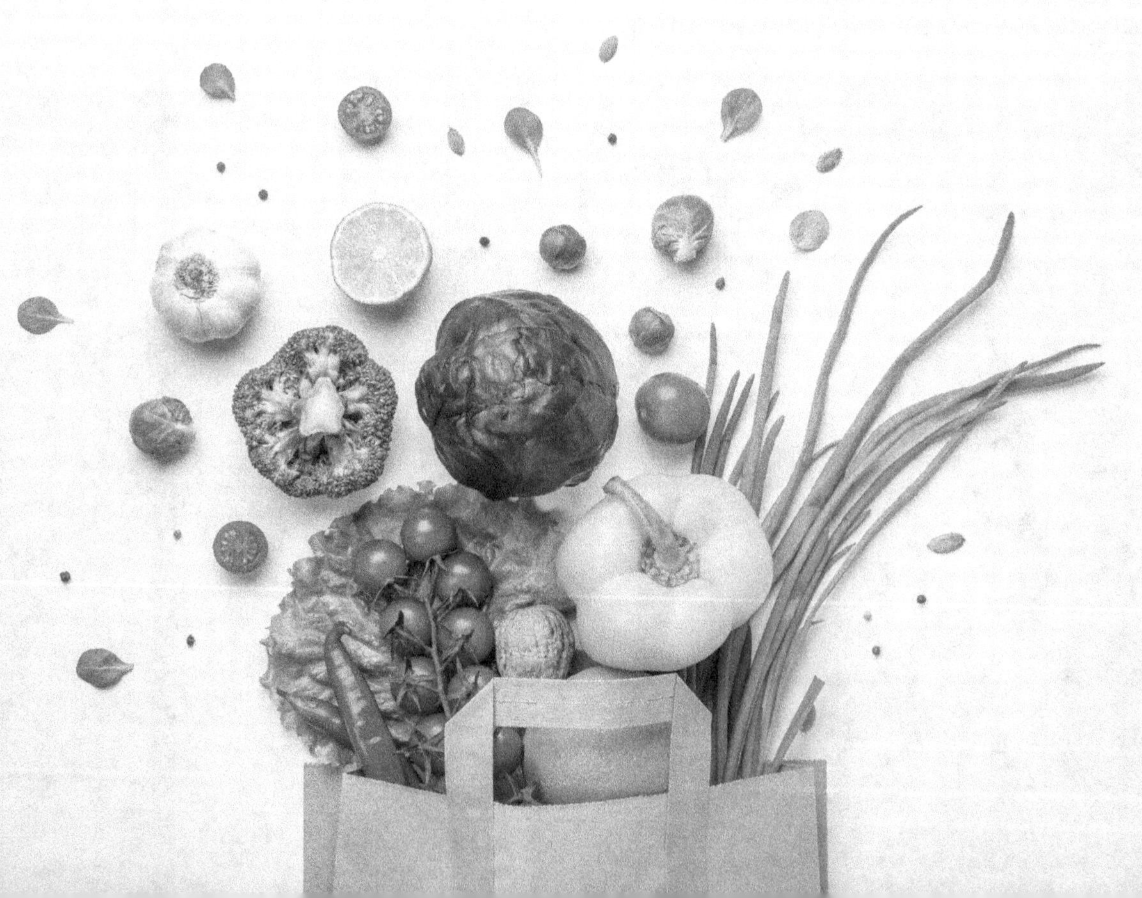

Snacks

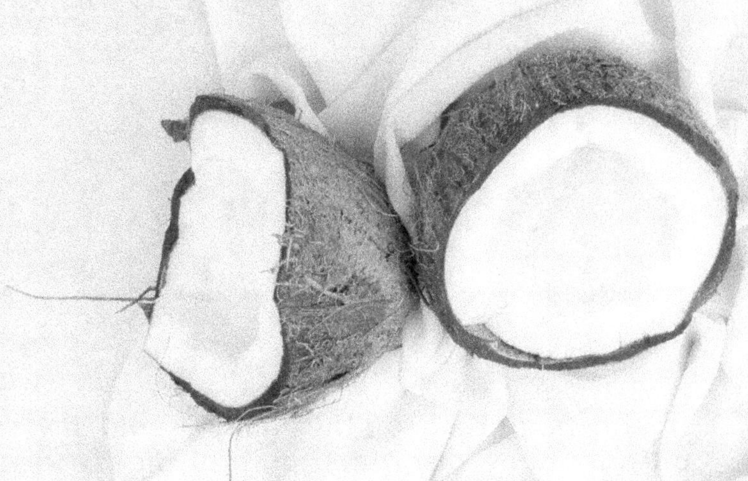

Energy balls with Seeds

Serving Size: 2
Serving size: 60 g or 2 oz.
Preparation time 10 minutes

INGREDIENTS:
¼ cup ground sesame seeds (40 g)
2 tbsp. unsweetened desiccated/shredded coconut (45 g)
2 pitted medjool dates, roughly chopped
½ tsp. ground turmeric
½ tsp. ground cinnamon
1 tbsp. unsweetened cocoa powder

DIRECTIONS: Soak the dates in hot water for about 10 minutes before blending. Add the rest of ingredients in a food processor and blend it all. You may need to stop to scrape the sides down occasionally. Scoop out 1 teaspoon of the mixture at a time and roll into little balls.

NUTRITIONAL INFORMATION

Energy (calories): 182 kcal
Protein: 4.32g
Fat: 9.39 g
Carbohydrates: 25.37 g
Fiber: 5.2 g

Amaranth Pudding with Coconut

Servings: 1 serving
Serving size: 210 g or 7oz.
Preparation time 5 minutes
Cooking time 15 minutes

INGREDIENTS:
3 tbsp. amaranth (24 g), precooked
½ a cup unsweetened coconut milk
1 oz. unsweetened shredded coconut
1/8 tsp. salt
1 tbsp. cinnamon
1 date, chopped

DIRECTIONS: Cook amaranth according to the box instructions. Drain it if any liquid remains. Heat coconut milk and add cooked amaranth. Add rest of the ingredients and cook them until they combine. Serve hot or chilled.

NUTRITIONAL INFORMATION

Energy (calories): 182 kcal
Protein: 4.32g
Fat: 9.39 g
Carbohydrates: 25.37 g
Fiber: 5.2 g

WHAT IS POWER SHOT GREENS SUPERFOOD BLEND?

In the beginning of this book I told my story of how I healed myself from auto-immune disorders, painful digestive issues and how Power Shot Greens Superfood was born. It took several months and a determination to find the right ingredients and specific formula that helped me heal.

Since then, I have been very fortunate to be able to hear many wonderful testimonies from those who also have been helped by Power Shot Greens Superfood. Power Shot contains all the unique Superfoods that are in this book, lovingly blended to make it simple and easy for you to use daily.

MIX, SHAKE AND DRINK.

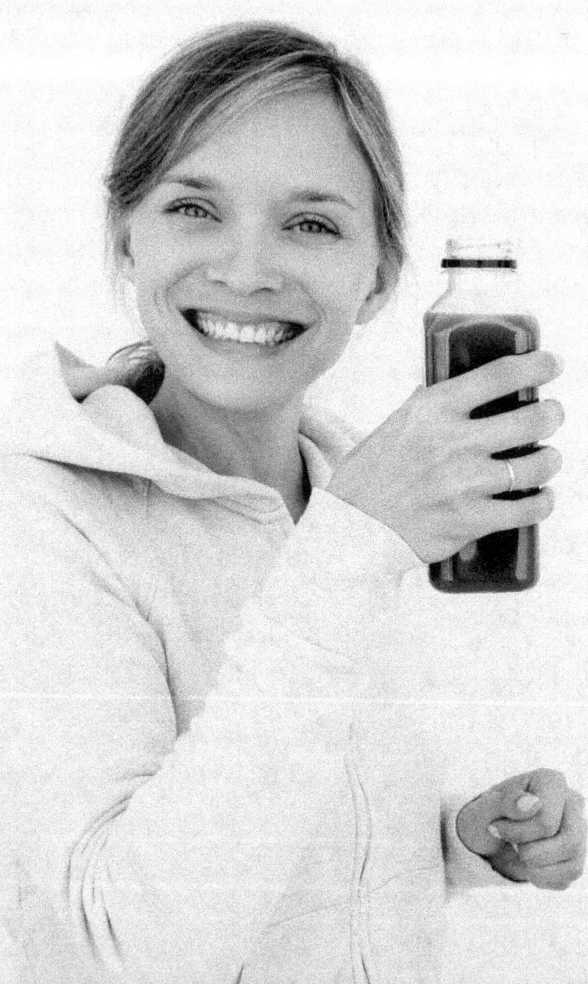

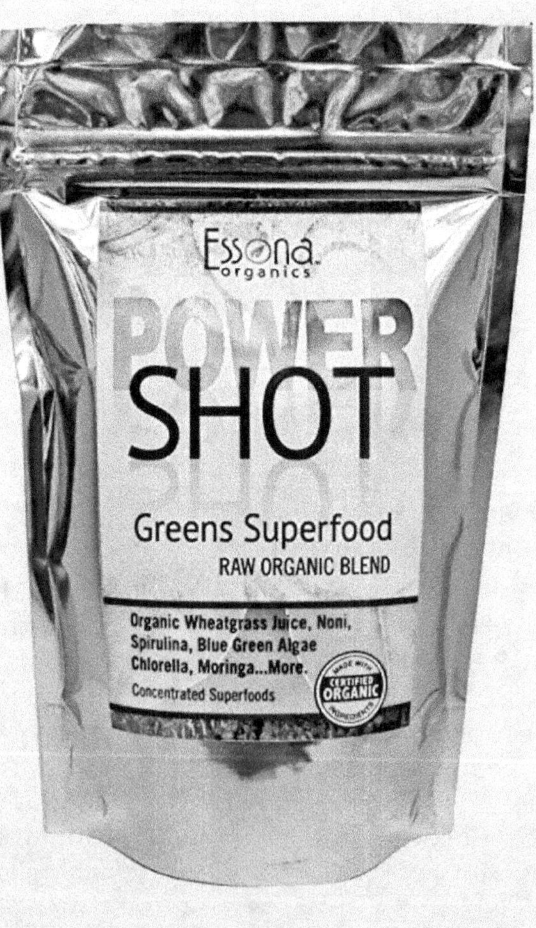

UNIQUE SUPERFOOD INGREDIENTS

The unique Superfoods in Power Shot Greens Superfood blend are ingredients that are not usually readily available at your local supermarket. Even if you could find all of them, it would be extremely costly and time-consuming to get them together and blend them correctly. We have already done all the research and work for you!

SYNERGISTICALLY BLENDED

The unique, pure ingredients are blended in a specific proportion to ensure that you receive the maximum results. Synergy means that the whole is greater than the sum of its parts.

NO FILLERS

There are absolutely no fillers in Power Shot Greens Superfood. Each ingredient is carefully chosen to provide a specific benefit and to work together in harmony with all the other ingredients.

60 DAY SUPPLY

Because there are no fillers, this 180 gram re-sealable pouch provides 60 servings at the nominal dose.

READILY DIGESTIBLE

Because the ingredients are in their purest form, they are readily available and highly absorbable by your body, so there is no waste.

TASTES GOOD

Power Shot Greens Superfood has been specially formulated to taste good and mix thoroughly and easily with water, juices or in a smoothie. Good taste means that you will look forward to using it daily.

USE DAILY

When added to your daily regimen, the results are noticeable and cumulative. The longer you use it, the better your results. You can be creative and use them in many ways – in smoothies, juices, water. Do not use in hot beverages like coffee or tea as the hot water will neutralize the natural enzyme activity.

Other Uses for Power Shot Greens Superfood

BEAUTY

Can also be used as a nourishing facial mask. Cleanse face. Rinse. Mix a small amount of Power Shot Greens Superfood with water into a paste. Apply to face as a mask. Leave on face for 15 minutes. Rinse. See and feel the rejuvenating effect.

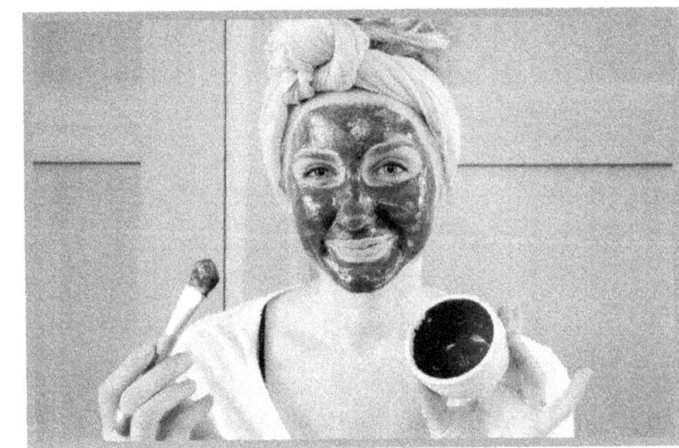

BODY

Poultice – Mix with a little water to a paste-like consistency. Apply to infected area. Cover with bandage.

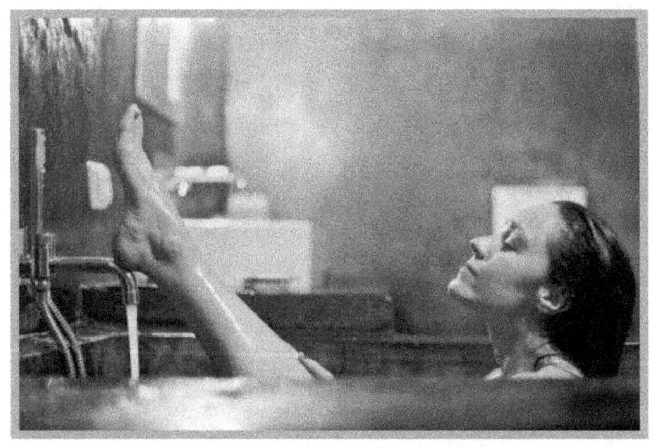

BATH

Sprinkle a few teaspoons into your bath water and experience a transforming Superfood Bath that is good for your skin. Your skin will drink in all the amazing vitamins, minerals and nutrients. You will see and feel the difference.

Testimonials – Happy Customers Speak Out

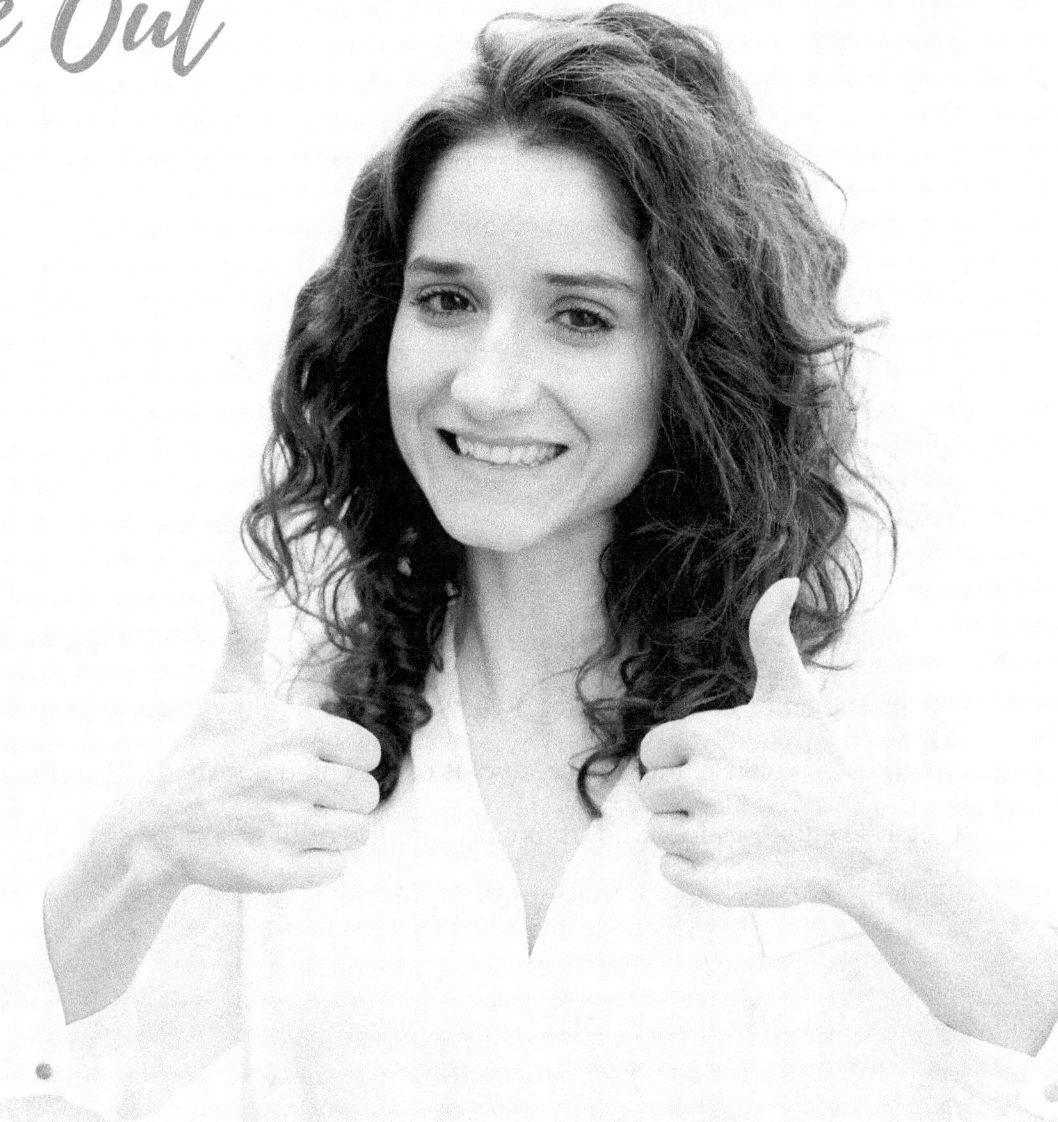

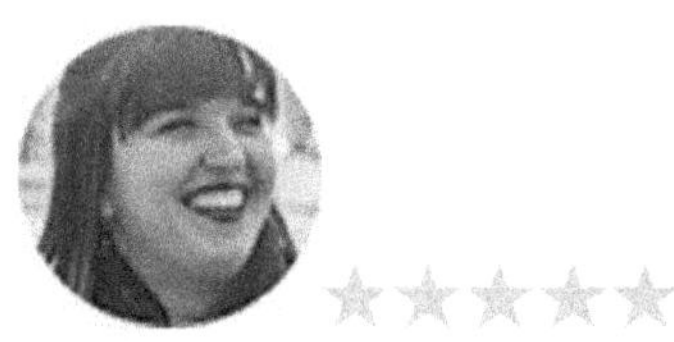

Kat H. I've tried a few greens including e3Live which is one of the best ones on the market... but this one, not only tastes the best, I can tell I'm detoxing because I started breaking out on my chest. I know most would think that's bad but it means it's cleansing my body and it will pass. I liked it so much that I decided to keep buying it even though it's no longer on sale. $36 for 2 months. Great deal & Good stuff!

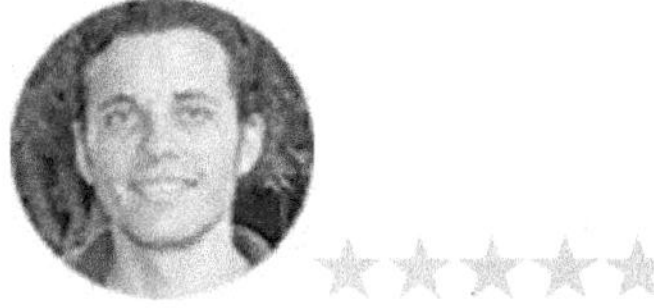

Mark M. I've worked in the supplement industry most of life and for the cost and profile of this product is great and simple. This is great tasting and chock full of the good stuff. My body is flying on this food. I normally just take moringa with my smoothies, but this just levelled up my smoothie making. Thank you for this product. Just amazing stuff here :)

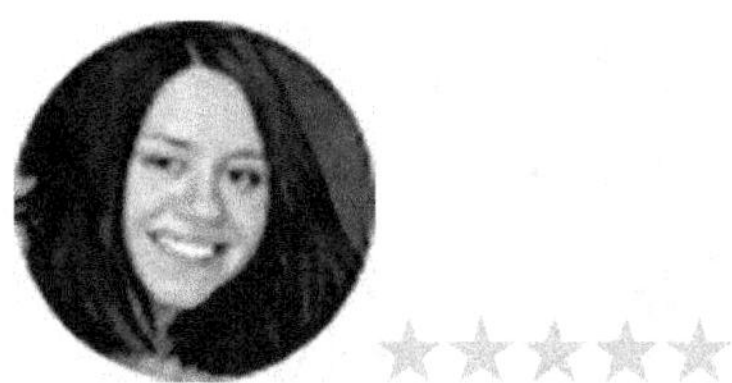

Michelle Queensborough I have been using this product for a few months now and I really like it. The color of the product is very rich and healthy looking and is a VERY vibrant blue green color. I believe that the product is of very high quality as it is pure (no chemicals added). I really like the product and assuming that the quality continues to remain consistently high, I will absolutely continue to reorder the product several times in the future.

Clean and good for you

Just finished my pack, about to order another one. I mean you can't go wrong with the ingredients. There are nothing in here that's bad for you. I just add this to my smoothies every morning.
Reviewed by: (Verified Buyer) Jay from Summit, NJ. on 1/21/2018

Five Stars

Excellent for my smoothie concoctions. Doesn't taste green. Great product!!!
Reviewed by: (Verified Buyer) Val from Tampa FL. on 4/3/2018

I LOVE this product

I LOVE this product. I put it in all my juices and smoothies. I have already recommend this product to my friends
Reviewed by: (Verified Buyer) Lydia from New York. on 12/28/2017

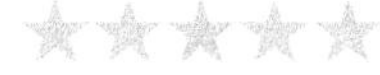

I reordered again because this isn't polluted with extra sugars or fruits, just good olde greens
Reviewed by: (Verified Buyer) William from Oregon. on 10/11/2017

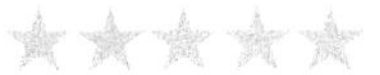

Five Stars

I love starting my day with these beautiful greens.
Reviewed by: (Verified Buyer) Janette from Salem. on 2/20/2018

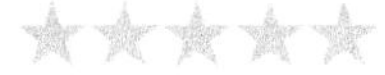

In LOVE with POWER SHOT

I LOVE this product! It is very healthy and I use this in my protein shake! I feel so much better use 1 tsp. Daily!
Reviewed by: (Verified Buyer) Laurie from Niagara Falls, NY. on 4/13/2018

Five Stars

Provides me with amazing energy!!!!!!!!!! Wow! I feel so healthy when I add it to my morning shake.
Reviewed by: (Verified Buyer) Maria from Charlotte, NC. on 12/11/2017

REVIEWS FROM AMAZON TOO!

Brian

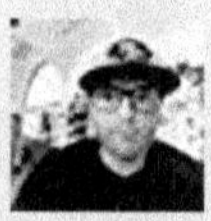

Alkalize your body!

April 4, 2017

Verified Purchase

Best greens I've tried, after about 2 months of taking habitually everyday started feeling really allot better no need for caffeine and in less pain, had a true alkalizing effect.

Jareth

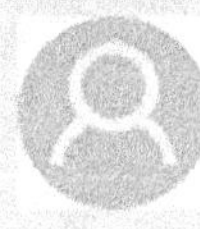

A great product that smells/tastes pretty good

February 5, 2018

Verified Purchase

A great product that smells/tastes pretty good. Always pop it in my morning smoothie or mix with some almond milk after a workout, ensuring I'm getting those somewhat obscure nutrients we vegans (and others) tend to miss out on. Definitely would recommend to anyone who wants a daily boost.

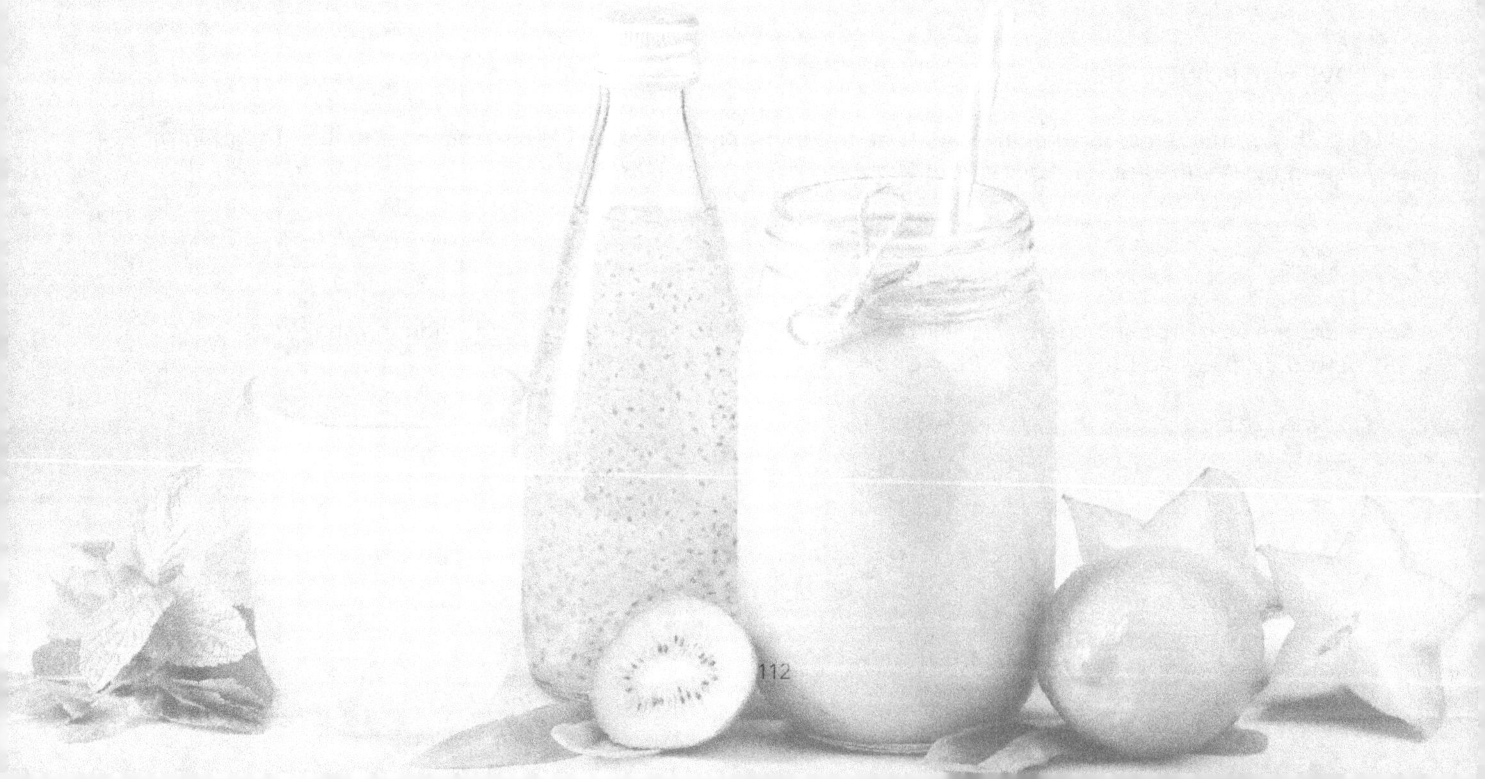

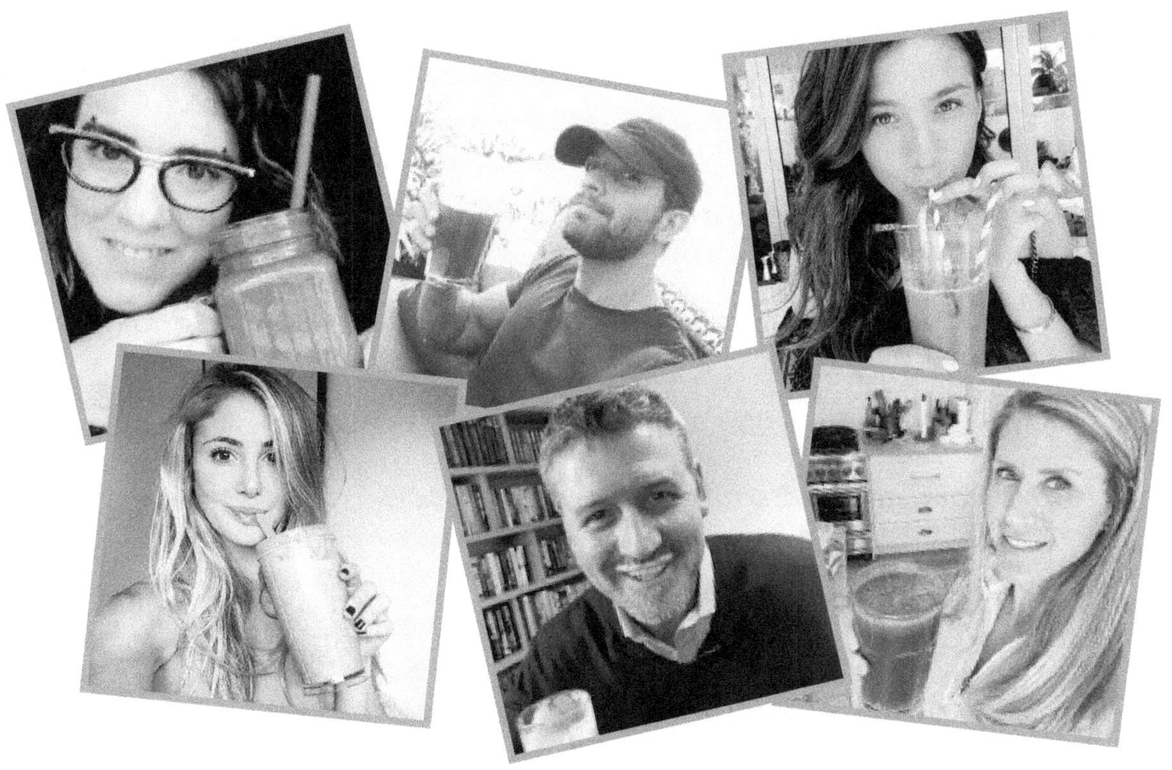

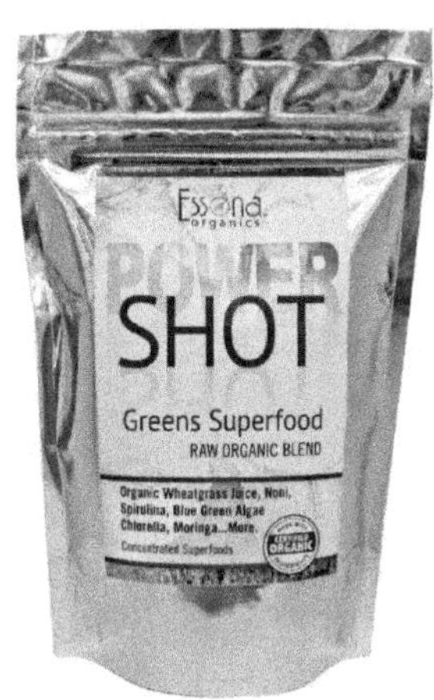

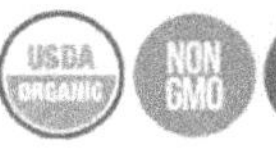

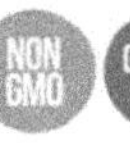

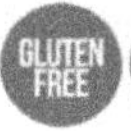

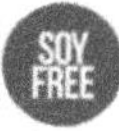

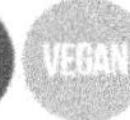

Please visit our website at www.essona.com for more info.

REFERENCES

https://blog.paleohacks.com/7-amazing-foods-that-cleanse-your-liver-naturally/

https://draxe.com/liver-function/

https://www.onegreenplanet.org/natural-health/cleaning-up-your-kidneys-helpful-foods-and-drinks-to-consider/

https://www.globalhealingcenter.com/natural-health/7-best-foods-support-kidney-function/

https://wellnessmama.com/35671/castor-oil-packs/

https://draxe.com/infrared-sauna/

https://wellnessmama.com/26717/dry-brushing-skin/

https://chopra.com/articles/the-benefits-of-tongue-scraping

https://gerson.org/gerpress/how-to-do-a-clay-pack/

http://healthbenefitsofwater.com/sea-salt-bath/

https://www.globalhealingcenter.com/natural-health/health-benefits-of-dandelion-root/

https://blog.paleohacks.com/8-herbs-that-detox-your-body-naturally/#

https://draxe.com/benefits-of-lemon-water/

https://draxe.com/milk-thistle-benefits/

https://helloglow.co/essential-oils-for-detox/

https://bodyecology.com/articles/a-minimalist-guide-to-the-detox-gene-plus-5-quick-detox-tips/

https://draxe.com/chlorophyll-benefits/